The Breathing Body's Biomechanics

Respiratory Mechanics And Anesthetic Implications For Optimal Pulmonary Function

Aella Storm

Contents

1 Introduction to Respiratory Physiology

The respiratory system, a marvel of biological engineering, ensures the continuous exchange of gases vital for life. Understanding its intricate workings is paramount, particularly for those involved in patient care, especially in situations where respiratory function might be compromised. This chapter provides a foundational understanding of respiratory physiology, essential for grasping the complexities discussed in subsequent chapters. We will explore the basic principles that govern breathing, laying the groundwork for more advanced concepts.

Efficient gas exchange relies on a precise interplay of mechanical processes, driven by the respiratory muscles. The diaphragm, a dome-shaped muscle separating the thoracic and abdominal cavities, plays a crucial role. Contraction of the diaphragm flattens it, increasing the volume of the thoracic cavity and decreasing intrapleural pressure, leading to lung expansion and air inhalation. Exhalation, generally passive, results from relaxation of the diaphragm and elastic recoil of the lungs. Accessory muscles, including intercostal muscles and abdominal muscles, become increasingly involved during strenuous activity or respiratory distress. Their recruitment adds to the inspiratory and expiratory efforts, expanding the capacity of the respiratory system to meet heightened oxygen demands.

Lung volumes and capacities represent key indicators of respiratory health. Tidal volume, the volume of air moved during a single breath, provides a measure of the normal breathing pattern. Inspiratory reserve volume, the additional air inhaled beyond a normal breath, and expiratory reserve volume, the extra air exhaled following a normal breath, quantify the respiratory reserve. Residual volume, the air remaining in the lungs after maximal exhalation, ensures continuous gas exchange even between breaths. The sum of these individual volumes constitutes the total lung capacity, reflecting the overall respiratory capacity. Understanding these volumes and capacities allows for the precise interpretation of pulmonary function tests, providing invaluable diagnostic insights. These measurements are crucial for assessing the overall health of the respiratory system, determining disease severity, and guiding treatment strategies.

The mechanics of breathing are governed by pressure gradients. The process begins with the creation of a negative pressure within the pleural space, the space surrounding the lungs. This negative pressure is vital for lung expansion and efficient gas exchange, pulling the lungs outwards towards the chest wall. Changes in pleural pressure drive the expansion and contraction of the lungs, driving the movement of air. Alterations in these pressures due to disease or injury can significantly impair respiratory function. Understanding these pressure relationships is central to appreciating the delicate balance required for efficient respiration. Precise regulation of these pressures is paramount for optimal respiratory function, which makes their importance for patient assessment and management even greater.

Airway resistance and lung compliance are intertwined factors influencing the efficiency of gas exchange. Airway resistance refers to the opposition to airflow within the respiratory tract, primarily determined by the diameter of the airways. Bronchoconstriction, as seen in asthma, significantly increases resistance, hindering airflow. Lung compliance reflects the elasticity of the lungs, representing their ability to expand in response to pressure changes. Conditions like pulmonary fibrosis reduce compliance, making breathing difficult. The interplay of these two factors influences the work of breathing, directly impacting the overall respiratory efficiency. Clinicians must carefully consider both when assessing and managing respiratory conditions, as it's this combination that is crucial in respiration's efficiency. These two aspects of respiratory function are closely related and profoundly impact the patient's overall health.

The intricacies of respiratory physiology are vast and complex, reaching beyond the scope of this introductory chapter. However, the fundamentals outlined here provide a solid foundation for understanding the subsequent chapters. A thorough grasp of basic respiratory mechanics, lung volumes, and the interplay of airway resistance and lung compliance are crucial for the proper interpretation of pulmonary function assessments and the management of respiratory complications. This understanding forms the basis of effective respiratory support and management within the context of anesthesia and surgery, as we will explore further in this book.

1.1 Basic Respiratory Mechanics

The process of breathing, seemingly effortless, involves a complex interplay of mechanics and physiology. Understanding these basics is paramount for anyone working within the respiratory field, from assessing a patient's baseline function to managing respiratory complications during and after anesthesia. Consider the act of inhalation: the diaphragm, a powerful muscle, contracts, flattening and descending. This increases the volume of the thoracic cavity, reducing pressure within. Consequently, air rushes into the lungs to equalize the pressure difference between the atmosphere and the alveoli—the tiny air sacs where gas exchange occurs. Expiration, conversely, involves relaxation of the diaphragm and intercostal muscles, reducing thoracic volume and increasing pressure, forcing air out of the lungs. This seemingly simple cycle is the foundation upon which the entire respiratory system functions.

These mechanics are significantly influenced by the physical properties of the lungs and the surrounding structures. Lung compliance, a measure of the lung's stretchability, describes how easily the lungs expand in response to pressure changes. A high compliance indicates easy expansion, while a low compliance suggests stiffness, hindering efficient ventilation. Airway resistance, another crucial factor, refers to the opposition to airflow within the respiratory tract. Narrowed airways, such as those seen in asthma, significantly increase resistance, demanding greater effort from the respiratory muscles to achieve adequate ventilation. Therefore, assessing compliance and resistance is vital for understanding a patient's overall respiratory status.

Further complicating the picture are the various accessory muscles involved in breathing. While the diaphragm and intercostal muscles perform the majority of the work during quiet breathing, forceful inspiration or expiration may recruit additional muscles, including the sternocleidomastoid, scalenes, and abdominal muscles. The engagement of these accessory muscles signals increased respiratory effort, often indicating underlying respiratory distress. Observing their involvement during physical examination is essential in determining the severity of respiratory compromise. For example, a patient struggling to breathe may exhibit obvious use of accessory muscles, suggesting underlying pathology such as COPD or pneumonia. Clinicians must meticulously monitor the utilization of these muscles during physical assessments.

Understanding pressure relationships within the respiratory system is equally crucial. Intrapleural pressure, the pressure within the pleural space—the space between the lungs and the chest wall—is normally negative relative to atmospheric pressure. This negative pressure is essential for keeping the lungs inflated. Changes in intrapleural pressure, either through disease or mechanical means like ventilation, directly impact lung volume and airflow. Likewise, alveolar pressure, the pressure within the alveoli, fluctuates during the respiratory cycle, driving air movement. These pressure gradients are vital components of efficient gas exchange, as they govern the flow of air into and out of the lungs. Accurate monitoring of these pressures is crucial especially in the context of anesthesia.

The act of breathing, while fundamental, is finely controlled by a complex network of neural and chemical signals. The respiratory center in the brainstem rhythmically generates the respiratory pattern, modulating the activity of the respiratory muscles. Peripheral chemoreceptors, located in the carotid and aortic bodies, continuously monitor blood gases (oxygen and carbon dioxide) and pH, sending signals to the respiratory center to adjust ventilation as needed. This feedback loop ensures that adequate oxygen is supplied and carbon dioxide is removed, maintaining homeostasis. Moreover, central chemoreceptors, located in the brainstem, monitor cerebrospinal fluid pH, providing additional input to the respiratory control system. Understanding this intricate control system is crucial when managing patients whose respiratory function is altered by disease, injury, or anesthetic agents.

Consider the interplay between ventilation and perfusion, two essential processes in gas exchange. Ventilation refers to the delivery of air to the alveoli, while perfusion refers to the flow of blood through the pulmonary capillaries surrounding the alveoli. An optimal balance between ventilation and perfusion is vital for efficient gas exchange. If ventilation is compromised in a particular region of the lung, but blood flow remains normal (ventilation-perfusion mismatch), that region will not contribute effectively to oxygen uptake and carbon dioxide removal. Conversely, if blood flow is reduced but ventilation remains normal, blood leaving the lungs will be poorly oxygenated. These mismatches can significantly impair gas exchange, leading to hypoxemia (low blood oxygen) and hypercapnia (high blood carbon dioxide). Therefore, understanding the complex interplay between ventilation and perfusion is critical for interpreting arterial blood gas results and effectively managing respiratory dysfunction. Such knowledge is essential for optimizing anesthetic techniques and preventing potentially lethal complications.

Finally, the efficient transport of gases within the body depends on several factors, notably hemoglobin's affinity for oxygen. Oxygen binds to hemoglobin in the lungs, forming oxyhemoglobin, which is then transported throughout the body. At the tissue level, oxygen dissociates from hemoglobin, allowing it to diffuse into the cells. Carbon dioxide, a waste product of cellular metabolism, diffuses from the tissues into the blood, where it is transported in various forms—dissolved in plasma, bound to hemoglobin, or as bicarbonate ions. Factors such as pH, temperature, and partial pressures of oxygen and carbon dioxide influence the affinity of hemoglobin for oxygen, affecting its ability to load and unload oxygen in the lungs and tissues respectively. Grasping these factors, critical for understanding oxygen transport and delivery, is fundamental for effective clinical management.

1.2 Lung Volumes and Capacities

Understanding lung volumes and capacities is fundamental to assessing respiratory function. These measurements, obtained through spirometry, provide a detailed picture of a patient's ability to inhale and exhale air. Tidal volume (TV), the volume of air moved in and out during a normal breath, represents the most immediate measure of respiratory function, directly reflecting the efficiency of each breathing cycle. Changes in tidal volume can signal early signs of respiratory compromise, necessitating closer monitoring and potential intervention.

Vital capacity (VC), encompassing tidal volume plus inspiratory reserve volume (IRV) and expiratory reserve volume (ERV), signifies the maximum amount of air a person can exhale after a maximal inhalation. This measurement provides a comprehensive assessment of lung function, encompassing the ability to both fully inhale and forcefully exhale. Reduced VC indicates diminished lung expansion or airway obstruction, potentially pointing to underlying respiratory pathology. Clinicians often use this value to monitor disease progression or treatment response.

Inspiratory reserve volume (IRV) represents the additional air inhaled beyond a normal breath. This reflects the capacity of the lungs to expand beyond their resting state. A decreased IRV may suggest restrictive lung disease, where lung expansion is physically limited. Conversely, an increased IRV can potentially indicate compensatory mechanisms for other underlying conditions. Understanding these dynamics is key to differentiating between various respiratory ailments. Careful interpretation of IRV, in conjunction with other lung volume measures, enables a more precise diagnostic evaluation.

Expiratory reserve volume (ERV) represents the additional air exhaled beyond a normal breath. It reflects the ability of the lungs to fully deflate. Decreased ERV often points to airway obstruction, commonly seen in obstructive pulmonary diseases like asthma or chronic obstructive pulmonary disease (COPD), or may signal increased airway resistance. Monitoring ERV changes can provide valuable insights into disease severity and response to treatment.

Residual volume (RV) refers to the air remaining in the lungs after a maximal exhalation. This air cannot be voluntarily expelled and plays a role in maintaining lung structure and preventing alveolar collapse. While not directly measurable with standard spirometry, RV can be estimated using various techniques, providing important information about lung compliance and potential air trapping. Elevated RV is a strong indicator of air trapping in obstructive lung diseases.

Total lung capacity (TLC) represents the sum of all lung volumes, including RV. This represents the maximum volume of air the lungs can hold. TLC changes are indicative of overall lung size and functionality. Reduced TLC suggests restrictive lung disease or other conditions limiting lung expansion, whereas increased TLC may indicate air trapping in obstructive diseases. Monitoring TLC fluctuations provides a comprehensive assessment of pulmonary capacity.

Functional residual capacity (FRC) refers to the amount of air remaining in the lungs after a normal exhalation. It represents the equilibrium point between the inward elastic recoil of the lungs and the outward recoil of the chest wall. FRC plays a critical role in gas exchange, as it contributes significantly to the alveolar ventilation and provides a reserve for oxygen exchange during periods of increased metabolic demand. Changes in FRC are often significant in various respiratory pathologies.

Inspiratory capacity (IC), the sum of tidal volume and inspiratory reserve volume, represents the maximum amount of air that can be inhaled after a normal exhalation. Reduced IC often signifies restrictive lung disease, limiting the lungs' ability to expand fully. This may stem from reduced lung compliance, increased chest wall rigidity, or neuromuscular weakness impacting respiratory muscles. Close observation of IC changes is vital for disease management.

Forced expiratory volume in one second (FEV1) and forced vital capacity (FVC) are important dynamic lung volumes that gauge the expiratory flow rate. FEV1 reflects the volume of air forcibly exhaled in one second after a maximal inhalation. FVC reflects the maximum amount of air that can be forcefully exhaled after a maximal inhalation. The ratio of FEV1/FVC is a key indicator of airway obstruction. A reduced ratio, often below 70%, suggests obstructive lung disease. These measurements are crucial for diagnosing and monitoring conditions such as asthma and COPD.

Understanding these lung volumes and capacities, along with their interrelationships, is crucial for interpreting spirometry results accurately. It facilitates the identification of respiratory impairments and guides appropriate clinical interventions. Precise measurement and interpretation of these parameters are paramount for effective respiratory care and the safe administration of anesthesia, helping clinicians assess risk, guide treatment, and ultimately optimize pulmonary function in patients. Further, monitoring these values throughout the treatment process provides continuous evaluation of the effectiveness of implemented therapies and the patient's respiratory status. Remember, this information represents an introductory overview; detailed understanding requires specialized training and practical experience.

2 Mechanics of Breathing

The diaphragm, a dome-shaped muscle separating the chest and abdomen, is the primary muscle of inspiration. Its contraction flattens the dome, increasing the vertical dimension of the thoracic cavity. Simultaneously, the external intercostal muscles, located between the ribs, contract, elevating the ribs and sternum, further expanding the chest cavity. This coordinated action creates a negative pressure within the lungs, drawing air inward. Expiration, in quiet breathing, is largely passive, relying on the elastic recoil of the lungs and chest wall. As these structures return to their resting position, air is expelled.

During more strenuous activities or when increased ventilation is needed, accessory muscles come into play. These include the sternocleidomastoid muscles in the neck, which elevate the sternum, and the scalene muscles, which lift the upper ribs. The abdominal muscles, particularly the rectus abdominis, internal and external obliques, and transversus abdominis, actively contract during forced expiration, compressing the abdominal contents and pushing the diaphragm upward, forcefully expelling air. Understanding the precise interplay of these muscles is vital for interpreting respiratory patterns and identifying potential dysfunction.

Pressure-volume relationships govern the mechanics of breathing. The lungs' compliance, or distensibility, refers to their ability to expand in response to changes in pressure. High compliance signifies easy expansion, while low compliance indicates stiffness and reduced expansibility. Factors influencing compliance include lung tissue elasticity, surface tension within the alveoli, and the presence of any restrictive lung disease. Airway resistance, the opposition to airflow, is primarily determined by airway diameter. Bronchoconstriction, as seen in asthma, significantly increases resistance, while bronchodilation decreases it. Both compliance and resistance critically affect the work of breathing.

Efficient gas exchange depends on the balance between ventilation (airflow) and perfusion (blood flow) in the lungs. Ventilation-perfusion (V/Q) matching ensures that well-ventilated alveoli are also adequately perfused with blood, maximizing oxygen uptake and carbon dioxide removal. Regional variations in V/Q exist in the upright lung, with the apices being relatively better ventilated than perfused, and the bases better perfused than ventilated. Diseases such as pneumonia and pulmonary embolism can severely disrupt V/Q matching, leading to impaired gas exchange and hypoxia.

Precise measurement of respiratory mechanics provides valuable insights into pulmonary function. Spirometry, a non-invasive technique, measures lung volumes and flows, assessing compliance and airway resistance. Pressure-volume loops, generated through sophisticated equipment, provide a graphical representation of lung mechanics, revealing subtle changes not easily detected by simpler methods. These advanced techniques enable a comprehensive assessment of respiratory health, crucial for managing various respiratory disorders and optimizing perioperative care.

Furthermore, understanding the subtle variations in respiratory patterns is critical. Changes in breathing rate, depth, and rhythm can indicate underlying respiratory distress or disease. Tachypnea (rapid breathing), bradypnea (slow breathing), and dyspnea (difficult or labored breathing) are common clinical presentations that necessitate careful evaluation. Auscultation, or listening to lung sounds with a stethoscope, can identify abnormal breath sounds like wheezes, crackles, or rhonchi, offering clues to the nature of respiratory compromise. Proper interpretation of these clinical findings is paramount for accurate diagnosis and timely intervention.

The mechanics of breathing are not just a passive process, but a complex interplay of muscular activity, pressure gradients, and anatomical structures. This integrated system, constantly adapting to physiological demands and environmental conditions, is fundamental to life itself. Any impairment within this system, regardless of the cause, can significantly impact overall health and quality of life. Thorough comprehension of these intricate mechanics, therefore, is critical for clinicians across various medical specialties. This knowledge provides a foundation for accurate diagnosis, effective treatment, and optimized patient care. A deeper understanding facilitates a more holistic approach to patient assessment, ensuring individualized care plans that address the specific respiratory needs of each individual. This is not just about understanding the mechanics; it's about applying that knowledge to enhance patient outcomes.

Finally, remember that the information provided here forms a foundational understanding of respiratory mechanics. Continuous learning and staying updated with advancements in the field are essential for any healthcare professional dealing with respiratory issues. The field is constantly evolving, with new research shedding light on the complexities of breathing and its implications for overall health. Therefore, engaging in continuing education and professional development is vital to provide the best possible care. This ongoing learning process will ensure that your knowledge remains current, allowing you to accurately assess, diagnose, and treat respiratory problems with confidence and expertise. The future of healthcare relies on this continual pursuit of knowledge and the commitment to providing the highest quality care.

2.1 The Respiratory Muscles

The diaphragm, a dome-shaped muscle separating the chest and abdomen, is the primary muscle of inspiration. Its contraction flattens the dome, increasing the vertical dimension of the thoracic cavity. This increase in volume decreases intrathoracic pressure, creating a negative pressure gradient that draws air into the lungs. Conversely, relaxation of the diaphragm allows the dome to rise, passively reducing the thoracic volume and expelling air. Understanding this fundamental mechanism is critical for comprehending normal breathing patterns and the impact of various patholo-

gies. Efficient diaphragmatic function is essential for optimal pulmonary function, and any impairment can significantly compromise ventilation.
External intercostal muscles, located between the ribs, play a crucial supporting role in inspiration. Their contraction elevates the ribs, increasing the anteroposterior and lateral dimensions of the thorax. This action further expands the thoracic cavity, augmenting the effect of diaphragm contraction. The interplay between diaphragm and intercostal muscles contributes to the overall efficiency of the breathing process, ensuring adequate lung inflation and efficient gas exchange. Weakness or paralysis of these muscles can drastically reduce inspiratory capacity, leading to respiratory distress.
Internal intercostal muscles are primarily expiratory muscles. Unlike the external intercostals, their contraction depresses the ribs, reducing thoracic volume. This action increases intrathoracic pressure, facilitating passive expiration. However, during forceful expiration, other muscles such as the abdominal muscles are also recruited. Their contraction increases intra-abdominal pressure, pushing the diaphragm upward and further compressing the lungs, thus enhancing the expiratory force. This coordinated muscle activity is critical for maintaining adequate ventilation, particularly during physical exertion or respiratory compromise.
Accessory muscles of respiration become active during increased respiratory demands, such as exercise or respiratory distress. These muscles include the sternocleidomastoid, scalene, and trapezius muscles in the neck and upper chest. Their contraction further elevates the ribs and sternum, significantly increasing thoracic volume. Recruitment of these accessory

muscles often indicates respiratory difficulty, and observing their use can be a valuable clinical indicator of the severity of respiratory compromise. Their involvement suggests the body is working harder to achieve adequate ventilation.

The mechanics of respiratory muscle function are intricate and involve complex neural control. The phrenic nerve innervates the diaphragm, while intercostal nerves innervate the intercostal muscles. These nerves receive signals from respiratory centers in the brainstem, which regulate the rate and depth of breathing based on various factors such as blood gas levels and metabolic demands. Understanding this neural control is essential for comprehending the effects of various medical conditions and anesthetic agents on respiratory function. Dysfunction within this complex neuro-muscular system can have far-reaching consequences on ventilation.

Respiratory muscle strength and endurance are crucial factors influencing respiratory function. Weakness of the respiratory muscles, which can result from various factors including neuromuscular diseases, prolonged bed rest, or critical illness, leads to reduced inspiratory capacity and increased work of breathing. Measuring respiratory muscle strength through techniques like maximal inspiratory pressure (MIP) and maximal expiratory pressure (MEP) provides valuable clinical information about the patient's respiratory status. Monitoring these parameters is crucial in assessing the need for respiratory support.

Optimal pulmonary function relies heavily on the efficient coordination and strength of the respiratory muscles. Any compromise in their function can have significant implications for gas exchange, oxygenation, and overall respiratory health. Therefore, a thorough understanding of respiratory muscle mechanics, innervation, and assessment techniques is crucial for clinicians involved in the care of patients with respiratory conditions. This knowledge is essential in providing appropriate respiratory support, optimizing anesthetic management, and promoting efficient postoperative recovery. Moreover, it underscores the importance of preventive measures to maintain respiratory muscle strength and function.

2.2 Pressure-Volume Relationships

The relationship between pressure and volume within the respiratory system is fundamental to understanding how we breathe. Think of the lungs as elastic balloons; their expansion and contraction are driven by pressure changes. Inspiration, or inhalation, begins with the diaphragm contracting and flattening, increasing the volume of the thoracic cavity. This increase in volume leads to a decrease in intrathoracic pressure, creating a pressure gradient that draws air into the lungs. Conversely, expiration, or exhalation, involves relaxation of the diaphragm and other respiratory muscles, decreasing the thoracic cavity volume and increasing intrathoracic pressure, forcing air out of the lungs. This simple interplay of pressure and volume is, however, significantly more complex in practice.

Compliance, a measure of the lung's distensibility, influences the pressure-volume relationship. Lungs with high compliance inflate easily with minimal pressure change, while those with low compliance require greater pressure for the same volume change. This compliance is affected by various factors, including lung tissue elasticity, surface tension within the alveoli, and the presence of any restrictive lung disease. For instance, conditions like pulmonary fibrosis reduce lung compliance, requiring significantly more respiratory effort for adequate ventilation. Understanding a patient's lung compliance is critical in assessing their respiratory status and guiding appropriate anesthetic management.

Airway resistance also plays a crucial role. The movement of air through the airways is not frictionless; resistance to airflow depends on several factors, including airway diameter and the viscosity of the air. Narrowed airways, as seen in asthma or bronchospasm, increase resistance, making breathing more difficult. This increased resistance requires increased respiratory effort and potentially reduces the effectiveness of ventilation, even if lung compliance remains adequate. An anesthesiologist must carefully consider airway resistance when managing a patient's ventilation, especially during procedures that can trigger bronchospasm.

The pressure-volume curve, a graphical representation of the relationship between pressure and volume within the lungs, provides a valuable tool for assessing respiratory function. The curve's shape reflects lung compliance and airway resistance. A steep curve indicates high compliance, meaning the lungs inflate readily. A flatter curve, conversely, suggests low compliance, indicating that the lungs are stiff and difficult to inflate. Changes in the curve's shape can reflect the progression of disease or the effects of anesthetic agents. Clinicians use this tool to monitor the patient's respiratory mechanics and make informed decisions about anesthetic and ventilatory support.

Furthermore, the pressure-volume relationship is not static; it varies during different phases of the respiratory cycle. For example, during deep breaths, the lungs may expand beyond their normal capacity, reaching higher volumes at increased pressures. Conversely, during shallow breaths, the lungs operate within a smaller portion of the pressure-volume curve. This dynamic relationship emphasizes the importance of considering the full range of respiratory effort when assessing a patient's respiratory status. Moreover, this dynamic aspect is critical when determining appropriate ventilatory support during anesthesia, where the goal is to maintain adequate gas exchange.

The concept of functional residual capacity (FRC), the lung volume at the end of a normal expiration, is also tied directly to this relationship. FRC represents the balance point between the elastic recoil of the lungs and the chest wall. Factors affecting lung compliance or chest wall mechanics can alter FRC. A reduced FRC, for instance, might signify an underlying respiratory condition requiring further evaluation. Anesthesiologists must be aware of FRC as its manipulation can affect gas exchange and potentially lead to respiratory complications. Therefore, understanding the relationship between FRC and pressure-volume is crucial for optimal anesthetic management.

Finally, understanding the intricacies of pressure-volume relationships allows for a better appreciation of the physiological challenges posed by various respiratory diseases. Conditions like restrictive lung diseases decrease compliance, requiring increased respiratory effort and potentially leading to respiratory fatigue. Obstructive lung diseases increase airway resistance, hindering effective ventilation. These pressure-volume changes are vital indicators of respiratory status, informing treatment strategies, and guiding anesthesia management. The ability to interpret and apply this knowledge to the clinical setting allows for a more precise and ultimately safer anesthetic experience for the patient. The skilled anesthetist leverages this knowledge to optimize ventilation and ensure adequate oxygenation during surgical procedures.

2.3 Airway Resistance and Compliance

Understanding airway resistance and compliance is crucial for comprehending the mechanics of breathing and their implications for anesthesia. Airway resistance, the opposition to airflow within the airways, primarily depends on airway diameter. Smaller airways, like those found in asthma or during bronchoconstriction, significantly increase resistance, requiring greater inspiratory effort. Conversely, larger airways facilitate easier airflow, minimizing the work of breathing. This dynamic interplay between airway size and resistance highlights the importance of maintaining patent airways.

Factors influencing airway resistance are numerous and complex, extending beyond simple diameter changes. Turbulent airflow, particularly at branching points within the airway tree, adds to resistance. Secretions within the airways, such as mucus, further obstruct airflow, amplifying resistance. Even the physical properties of the airways themselves—their elasticity and compliance—contribute to the overall resistance. Clinicians must carefully consider these multifaceted influences when assessing and managing patients. For instance, in patients with cystic fibrosis, the thick, sticky mucus significantly increases airway resistance, making ventilation challenging.

Airway compliance, on the other hand, reflects the lungs' distensibility—their ability to expand in response to pressure changes. A highly compliant lung expands easily with minimal pressure, indicating healthy elasticity. Conversely, low compliance indicates stiff lungs, requiring substantial pressure to achieve adequate inflation. This decreased distensibility may result from conditions like pulmonary fibrosis, where the lung tissue becomes scarred and less elastic, or acute respiratory distress syndrome (ARDS), where fluid buildup in the alveoli impairs lung expansion.

Assessing both airway resistance and compliance is integral to evaluating respiratory function. Various tools and techniques are available, from simple clinical examinations like auscultation to sophisticated techniques like spirometry and whole-body plethysmography. Clinicians use these assessments to identify underlying respiratory issues, offering valuable insights into the patient's overall respiratory health. The information obtained helps guide treatment strategies, from bronchodilators to mechanical ventilation support, optimizing respiratory function.

The relationship between airway resistance and compliance is not merely additive. Their combined effect on the work of breathing is significant, influencing the patient's comfort, respiratory drive, and ability to maintain adequate oxygenation. For instance, increased airway resistance necessitates greater inspiratory effort, potentially leading to fatigue and respiratory muscle exhaustion. Reduced compliance compounds this problem, increasing the pressure required for adequate lung inflation, further exacerbating the respiratory workload. In clinical settings, a patient with both high resistance and low compliance faces a substantial challenge in maintaining adequate ventilation.

Anesthesia further complicates the equation. Many anesthetic agents depress respiratory drive, potentially masking subtle changes in airway resistance and compliance. This necessitates vigilant monitoring and proactive management to prevent respiratory compromise. The use of neuromuscular blocking agents, while often necessary for surgical procedures, further decreases respiratory muscle strength and may impact the ability to compensate for increased airway resistance or decreased compliance. Therefore, meticulous respiratory monitoring is crucial throughout the perioperative period to detect and address any potential adverse changes.

Moreover, understanding airway resistance and compliance is not solely important for critical care situations. It holds significance for pre-operative assessment as well. For example, a patient with a history of asthma presents a higher risk of airway complications during and after surgery. A thorough pre-operative evaluation of both airway resistance and compliance helps clinicians anticipate potential respiratory challenges and develop appropriate management plans. This may include optimizing medication, performing bronchodilator treatments, or adopting different anesthetic techniques to minimize the risk of respiratory complications. In essence, understanding airway mechanics facilitates a safer and more successful surgical experience.

Finally, the principles of airway resistance and compliance extend beyond the immediate perioperative setting. Chronic respiratory diseases, such as chronic obstructive pulmonary disease (COPD), are characterized by persistently increased airway resistance and often altered lung compliance. Understanding these biomechanical factors is crucial for developing effective long-term management strategies. These strategies often involve optimizing medication, pulmonary rehabilitation, and lifestyle modifications to alleviate symptoms and improve overall quality of life. In conclusion, a comprehensive grasp of airway resistance and compliance provides a foundation for effective respiratory care, spanning from pre-operative assessment to post-operative recovery, and extending to the ongoing management of chronic respiratory conditions.

3 Gas Exchange and Transport

Efficient gas exchange relies heavily on the interplay between ventilation and perfusion. Ventilation, the movement of air into and out of the lungs, must be precisely matched with perfusion, the blood flow through the pulmonary capillaries. This matching, or V/Q matching, is crucial for optimal oxygen uptake and carbon dioxide removal. An imbalance, such as underperfusion (low V/Q) in a region of the lung, leads to inadequate oxygenation of that area's blood, while overperfusion (high V/Q) results in wasted ventilation because not all the inhaled oxygen is utilized. Clinical scenarios such as pulmonary embolism significantly impair V/Q matching, impacting oxygenation and necessitating prompt intervention.

Understanding alveolar gas equations is foundational to comprehending gas exchange. These equations, derived from principles of gas diffusion and partial pressures, allow us to calculate the partial pressures of oxygen and carbon dioxide in the alveoli. These alveolar partial pressures are essential because they directly influence the driving force for gas exchange across the alveolar-capillary membrane. Factors such as the inspired oxygen fraction (FiO2) and the respiratory quotient (RQ), reflecting the ratio of CO_2 produced to O_2 consumed, are key components of these calculations, helping us predict alveolar gas composition under various physiological conditions. Accurate estimations are pivotal in managing patients with respiratory compromise, such as those with hypoxemia.

Oxygen transport from the lungs to the tissues involves a complex process relying primarily on hemoglobin, the oxygen-carrying protein in red blood cells. Hemoglobin's affinity for oxygen is influenced by factors such as pH, temperature, and the partial pressure of carbon dioxide—the Bohr effect. A decrease in pH or an increase in temperature or PCO_2 lowers hemoglobin's oxygen affinity, facilitating oxygen unloading in the tissues. Conversely, a higher pH or lower temperature and PCO_2 increase affinity, promoting oxygen loading in the lungs. These dynamic interactions ensure efficient oxygen delivery to metabolically active tissues, highlighting the intricate regulatory mechanisms governing oxygen transport. Understanding these factors is crucial for managing patients with conditions affecting oxygen-carrying capacity.

Carbon dioxide transport, unlike oxygen, involves multiple pathways. A significant portion is transported as bicarbonate ions (HCO_3^-), formed by the hydration of CO_2 within red blood cells. This reaction is catalyzed by carbonic anhydrase. The resulting bicarbonate ions diffuse out of red blood cells into the plasma, helping buffer blood pH. A smaller fraction of CO_2 is dissolved directly in plasma, while another portion binds to hemoglobin. This multi-faceted approach reflects the body's efficiency in removing metabolic waste products, with the bicarbonate buffer system particularly vital in maintaining acid-base balance. A dysfunction in this system, as seen in respiratory acidosis, severely affects pH and necessitates prompt management.

Diffusion limitations in gas exchange can occur due to various factors. These factors impact the rate at which gases traverse the alveolar-capillary membrane. A thickened membrane, as in interstitial lung disease, or decreased surface area, as seen in emphysema, slows the diffusion of oxygen and carbon dioxide. Similarly, factors that decrease the driving pressure, such as hypoventilation or low alveolar PO2, also impede efficient gas exchange. In clinical settings, understanding these diffusion limitations is essential for interpreting arterial blood gas results and guiding appropriate interventions. For example, supplemental oxygen may be less effective in cases where diffusion limitations are significant.

The delicate balance between oxygen delivery and tissue consumption is crucial for maintaining adequate oxygenation. In normal physiology, this balance is tightly regulated. However, in disease states or during anesthesia, this balance can be disrupted. For instance, circulatory shock can severely limit tissue oxygen delivery even if alveolar oxygenation remains adequate. Similarly, increased metabolic demands, such as during exercise or fever, can increase tissue oxygen consumption, leading to potential hypoxia despite adequate delivery. Anesthetic agents can further complicate matters, directly impacting ventilation and oxygen transport capacity. Therefore, vigilant monitoring of oxygen saturation and tissue perfusion is critical, especially during periods of increased stress or disease. Understanding the potential disruptions to this balance allows for timely adjustments in treatment strategies to maintain optimal oxygenation and prevent hypoxia.

3.1 Alveolar Gas Equations

Understanding alveolar gas exchange is crucial for managing respiratory function, particularly in the context of anesthesia. Accurate calculation of alveolar partial pressures of oxygen (PAO2) and carbon dioxide (PACO2) allows for a precise assessment of ventilation and gas exchange efficiency. These calculations are vital in determining the adequacy of oxygenation and ventilation, especially in patients with compromised pulmonary function or those under the influence of anesthetic agents. Failure to appropriately manage these gases can lead to hypoxemia or hypercapnia, both with potentially serious consequences.

The alveolar gas equation, a cornerstone of respiratory physiology, offers a quantitative approach to estimating PAO2. This equation considers the inspired partial pressure of oxygen (PIO2), the partial pressure of water vapor (PH2O), and the respiratory exchange ratio (R), which reflects the ratio of carbon dioxide produced to oxygen consumed. While R is typically assumed to be 0.8, it can vary in specific clinical scenarios, such as during metabolic acidosis or during the administration of certain anesthetic agents; therefore precise measurements are vital. This variability emphasizes the importance of considering individual patient factors to refine the accuracy of the alveolar gas equation. A simple formula, PAO2 = PIO2

– (PACO2/R) – PH2O, illustrates the relationship between these variables. The equation clarifies how changes in any of these factors directly impact PAO2. This understanding is vital for interpreting arterial blood gas results and making informed clinical decisions.

Estimating PACO2, on the other hand, requires a different approach. Unlike PAO2, which is dependent on several variables, PACO2 is essentially a direct reflection of alveolar ventilation. This means accurately measuring PACO2 provides insights into the effectiveness of ventilation. However, we must remember that PACO2 is not equivalent to arterial PCO2(PaCO2), although they correlate closely. Factors such as ventilation-perfusion (V/Q) mismatch and diffusion limitations can lead to discrepancies. Thus, interpreting arterial blood gas analysis demands a comprehensive understanding beyond just the alveolar gas equation's direct results.

The clinical application of these equations extends beyond simple calculations. For instance, in patients undergoing surgery under general anesthesia, monitoring PAO2 and PACO2 helps clinicians detect and manage potential respiratory complications. The use of the alveolar gas equation allows for real-time assessment and adjustments to the anesthetic and ventilatory strategies. This ensures optimal gas exchange and avoids potentially detrimental hypoxemia or hypercapnia. The clinician can then use this information to make informed decisions, such as adjusting the inspired oxygen concentration, ventilator settings, or even the anesthetic agent being administered.

Furthermore, the alveolar gas equation aids in identifying specific pathophysiological processes. For example, a low PAO2 despite adequate ventilation can indicate shunt or diffusion impairment, while a high PACO2 implies inadequate alveolar ventilation. These equations, combined with other clinical data, aid in differentiating between various respiratory disorders and guiding appropriate interventions. This is critical for making early diagnoses and implementing effective treatment, improving patient outcomes. Accurate diagnosis leads to timely and effective interventions.

In summary, mastering the alveolar gas equations and their clinical applications is integral to the practice of respiratory medicine, especially in the context of anesthesia. This chapter has emphasized the significance of the PAO2 and PACO2 calculations. Understanding the interplay between these parameters and their correlation with arterial blood gas values enables clinicians to make informed decisions about patient management, leading to better outcomes. Careful consideration of individual patient factors such as age, body mass index, pre-existing conditions, and the specific anesthetic agents used must always inform the interpretation of these calculations. The equations provide a framework, but skilled clinical judgment is crucial for their proper utilization in providing optimal patient care. Remembering that these are estimates, and the actual values may vary, is essential to sound clinical practice. Thus, continuous monitoring and vigilant interpretation are paramount in ensuring optimal respiratory function in the perioperative setting. The equations themselves are tools; it is the clinician's knowledge and clinical judgment that transform them into effective agents for improved patient care.

3.2 Oxygen Transport

Oxygen, vital for life, doesn't simply dissolve passively into the blood; its transport is a sophisticated process involving hemoglobin, the iron-containing protein residing within red blood cells. Hemoglobin's remarkable structure – four subunits, each capable of binding one oxygen molecule – allows for cooperative binding. This means the binding of one oxygen molecule increases the affinity of the remaining subunits, facilitating efficient oxygen uptake in the lungs where partial pressure is high. Conversely, in tissues with lower oxygen partial pressure, the affinity decreases, promoting oxygen release to metabolically active cells. Factors such as pH, temperature, and 2,3-bisphosphoglycerate (2,3-BPG) influence hemoglobin's oxygen-binding affinity, subtly adjusting oxygen delivery based on tissue demands. Understanding this intricate interplay is critical for comprehending the body's oxygen supply mechanism.

A small fraction of oxygen, however, dissolves directly into plasma. While seemingly insignificant compared to hemoglobin-bound oxygen, dissolved oxygen plays a crucial role in establishing the partial pressure gradient driving oxygen movement from alveoli to blood. This dissolved oxygen contributes to the overall oxygen content of the blood, albeit a minor component compared to the oxygen bound to hemoglobin. The precise measurement of arterial blood oxygen content, reflecting both dissolved and bound oxygen, is essential in assessing a patient's oxygenation status and guiding clinical decisions. This emphasizes the integrated nature of the various oxygen transport methods working in concert.

The efficiency of oxygen transport depends heavily on several physiological factors. Cardiac output, determining the rate of blood flow to tissues, directly impacts oxygen delivery. A reduced cardiac output, as seen in various cardiovascular conditions, can lead to inadequate oxygen supply even if the oxygen saturation is normal. Similarly, the number of red blood cells, and thus the total hemoglobin concentration, significantly influences oxygen-carrying capacity. Anemia, characterized by reduced red blood cell count or hemoglobin levels, impairs oxygen transport, resulting in hypoxia. Proper diagnostic tools and laboratory tests are essential to assess these critical components of oxygen transport and identify any potential deficiencies.

Furthermore, the integrity of the alveolar-capillary membrane is paramount. This thin barrier facilitates efficient gas exchange; its thickening or damage, as seen in various lung diseases, hinders oxygen diffusion into the blood. Pathological processes can disrupt the delicate balance of this interface, impeding oxygen transfer and compromising tissue oxygenation. Understanding the physiological integrity of this membrane, therefore, provides valuable insights into potential disruptions and their impact on oxygen delivery. This aspect highlights the vulnerability of oxygen transport to underlying pathologies.

In clinical settings, assessing oxygen transport relies on multiple techniques. Pulse oximetry provides a non-invasive measure of arterial oxygen saturation, reflecting the percentage of hemoglobin bound to oxygen.

Arterial blood gas analysis offers a more comprehensive evaluation, providing precise measurements of partial pressures of oxygen and carbon dioxide, pH, and bicarbonate levels. These are crucial in determining the adequacy of oxygenation and ventilation. Careful interpretation of these diagnostic data helps clinicians understand the overall efficiency of oxygen transport and identify any underlying physiological impairments that may be present. Such evaluation is especially crucial in patients with compromised respiratory function or those under anesthesia where the respiratory system may be suppressed.

The interplay between oxygen transport and the anesthetic implications can be complex and requires careful consideration. Many anesthetic agents can depress respiratory function, indirectly impacting oxygen transport by decreasing ventilation and the partial pressure of oxygen in the alveoli. Additionally, some anesthetics can directly affect hemoglobin's affinity for oxygen. Monitoring and managing these interactions are critical in maintaining adequate oxygen delivery to tissues during surgical procedures. Understanding these subtleties allows for tailored anesthetic management, aiming to minimize adverse effects on oxygen transport.

Therefore, a comprehensive understanding of oxygen transport is fundamental for both the basic scientist and the clinician. From the molecular mechanisms of hemoglobin binding to the clinical assessment of oxygenation, understanding the intricacies of this process is essential for maintaining optimal respiratory function and patient well-being. This knowledge is particularly critical in situations involving respiratory compromise or during anesthetic management, where efficient oxygen delivery is paramount to a positive outcome. A clear comprehension of these processes is essential for making informed decisions in clinical practice, ultimately contributing to better patient care.

3.3 Carbon Dioxide Transport

Unlike oxygen, which primarily binds to hemoglobin, carbon dioxide transport is a multifaceted process involving three primary mechanisms: dissolved CO2, bicarbonate ions (HCO3-), and carbamino compounds. A small fraction, approximately 7%, dissolves directly into the plasma, contributing minimally to total transport but establishing a partial pressure gradient crucial for gas exchange. This dissolved CO2 is the driving force for the other transport mechanisms. Understanding these dynamics is essential for clinicians, especially in scenarios where respiratory function is compromised.

The majority of CO2 transport, roughly 70%, occurs as bicarbonate ions. Within red blood cells (RBCs), carbonic anhydrase, a remarkably efficient enzyme, catalyzes the rapid conversion of CO2 and water into carbonic acid (H2CO3). Carbonic acid subsequently dissociates into bicarbonate and hydrogen ions (H+). The bicarbonate ions then diffuse out of the RBCs into the plasma, while the hydrogen ions remain within the RBCs, influencing the oxygen-hemoglobin dissociation curve. This interplay is a key factor in the Bohr effect, which describes how pH changes affect hemoglobin's affinity for oxygen. In essence, the lower the pH (higher H+

concentration), the less effectively hemoglobin binds oxygen, facilitating oxygen release in tissues with high CO_2 production.

The remaining 23% of CO_2 is transported bound to proteins, notably hemoglobin, forming carbamino compounds. This binding primarily occurs at amino acid residues within the globin portion of the hemoglobin molecule, not at the heme groups responsible for oxygen binding. This crucial distinction allows for simultaneous transport of both gases, even with their different binding affinities and sites. However, the amount of CO_2 bound to hemoglobin is influenced by both CO_2 partial pressure and the degree of hemoglobin oxygen saturation. Therefore, changes in oxygen saturation can significantly affect CO_2 transport. Clinicians must consider these interactions when managing patients with respiratory or circulatory compromise.

The Haldane effect, another critical aspect of CO_2 transport, describes the impact of oxygen saturation on CO_2 carrying capacity. Specifically, deoxyhemoglobin (hemoglobin without bound oxygen) has a higher affinity for CO_2 than oxyhemoglobin (hemoglobin with bound oxygen). Consequently, in tissues with low oxygen tension, CO_2 loading onto hemoglobin is enhanced. Conversely, in the lungs, where oxygen levels are high, the release of oxygen from hemoglobin increases its capacity to bind to oxygen rather than CO_2, effectively unloading the CO_2 for exhalation. Mastering these principles is vital in understanding oxygen and CO_2 exchange.

Efficient CO_2 transport relies heavily on the integrity of the respiratory and circulatory systems. Any impairment, such as pulmonary embolism or cardiac failure, can significantly disrupt the equilibrium of gas transport. The resulting acidosis or hypercapnia can have profound systemic effects, leading to various clinical manifestations depending on the severity and duration of the disruption. Precise management depends on the underlying cause and requires careful monitoring of blood gases, pH, and other relevant parameters. Understanding the underlying mechanisms is key to effective clinical interventions.

The precise interplay between oxygen and carbon dioxide transport is far more intricate than often initially perceived. The intricate details of these processes highlight the delicate balance that sustains human life. It's a testament to the body's incredible adaptability that it can maintain this equilibrium even under stressful conditions. However, the limits of this adaptive capacity must be understood in clinical practice. This chapter, although concise, aims to provide a strong foundational knowledge that will enable clinicians to more effectively approach complex respiratory scenarios. The practical application of this knowledge is invaluable in patient care, from diagnostics to therapeutic interventions.

Furthermore, understanding the subtleties of CO2 transport provides crucial insight into the effectiveness of various anesthetic agents and their potential to disrupt this delicate balance. Certain anesthetics, for example, can suppress respiratory drive, leading to hypercapnia. Recognizing the impact of these effects allows for precise adjustments to anesthetic management, ultimately improving patient outcomes. It is crucial for anesthesiologists to master these principles, as they can significantly influence respiratory function during surgical procedures. A thorough understanding of this chapter is thus fundamental for safe and effective anesthesiology practice. The interactions are complex, but the reward of this knowledge for patient well-being is immeasurable.

In summary, understanding CO2 transport involves grasping its multifaceted nature. It is not a singular process, but rather a dynamic interplay of solubility, enzymatic reactions, and protein binding, all interwoven with oxygen transport and influenced by physiological factors. Clinical application of this knowledge proves invaluable in managing respiratory conditions, optimizing anesthetic practices, and ensuring successful patient outcomes. Continuous learning and refinement of this knowledge base is essential for continued improvement in healthcare. Mastering the principles discussed here provides an essential foundation for a deeper dive into more complex respiratory and anesthetic management.

Therefore, meticulous consideration of these detailed factors will enhance a clinician's ability to properly assess, diagnose, and treat patients presenting with respiratory compromise. Recognizing the interconnectedness of oxygen and CO2 transport, along with the Haldane and Bohr effects, will enhance the understanding of the body's response to disease or anesthetic intervention. This comprehension becomes essential for optimal management in various clinical settings. By appreciating the intricacies of CO2 transport, we can strive for better patient outcomes and an elevated standard of care. This detailed knowledge is not merely academic; it is a critical component of effective and compassionate clinical practice.

3.4 Ventilation-Perfusion Matching

Efficient gas exchange hinges on the precise matching of ventilation (V), the movement of air into and out of the alveoli, and perfusion (Q), the blood flow through the pulmonary capillaries surrounding those alveoli. An ideal V/Q ratio is approximately 1.0, ensuring that every alveolus receives a sufficient amount of air and blood for optimal oxygen uptake and carbon dioxide removal. Deviation from this ideal ratio, however, significantly impacts oxygenation and can lead to various respiratory complications.

Consider a scenario where ventilation is high but perfusion is low, leading to a high V/Q ratio (V/Q > 1). This situation, often encountered in pulmonary embolism or areas of lung collapse, results in wasted ventilation, as the alveoli are filled with air but not adequately perfused with blood to facilitate gas exchange. Oxygen enters the alveoli but doesn't efficiently transfer to the blood, and carbon dioxide removal is impaired. The net effect is hypoxemia, a low partial pressure of oxygen in the arterial blood.

Conversely, a low V/Q ratio (V/Q < 1) signifies areas where perfusion exceeds ventilation. This is commonly observed in conditions like pneumonia, where fluid accumulation in the alveoli obstructs airflow while blood flow continues. In this case, blood flows past poorly ventilated alveoli, resulting in a shunting effect. The blood entering the systemic circulation has lower-than-normal oxygen levels, leading to hypoxemia, and the impaired removal of carbon dioxide can result in hypercapnia. Both hypoxemia and hypercapnia can have profound systemic effects, affecting multiple organ systems and potentially leading to severe consequences.

The body utilizes various compensatory mechanisms to maintain adequate oxygen delivery despite V/Q mismatches. For example, hypoxemia triggers increased ventilation through chemoreceptor stimulation. The respiratory system attempts to improve the V/Q ratio by increasing ventilation to better match perfusion. However, these compensatory mechanisms are limited, and severe or widespread V/Q mismatches can overwhelm the body's ability to maintain normal oxygenation and carbon dioxide removal.

Understanding V/Q mismatches is crucial for clinicians, particularly anesthesiologists. During surgery, various factors can affect ventilation and perfusion, potentially leading to V/Q imbalances. For example, anesthesia itself can depress respiration, affecting ventilation. Furthermore, the surgical position, surgical procedures near the chest, or the administration of certain medications can also compromise ventilation and/or perfusion. Careful monitoring of respiratory parameters, such as arterial blood gases, pulse oximetry, and end-tidal carbon dioxide, is essential to detect and address potential V/Q mismatches intraoperatively.

Anesthesiologists must consider the patient's underlying lung conditions when planning anesthesia. Preoperative evaluation should include a thorough respiratory assessment, identifying patients at risk of developing V/Q imbalances. This might involve pulmonary function tests, chest imaging, and a comprehensive medical history. The choice of anesthetic agents, ventilation strategies, and postoperative respiratory management should be tailored to minimize the risk of V/Q mismatches and optimize postoperative pulmonary function.

Addressing V/Q mismatches often involves supportive measures aimed at improving ventilation and oxygenation. This may include supplemental oxygen therapy, mechanical ventilation with adjustments to respiratory rate, tidal volume, and positive end-expiratory pressure (PEEP), and bronchodilators to improve airway patency. In severe cases, interventions such as prone positioning or extracorporeal membrane oxygenation (ECMO) might be necessary to provide adequate oxygenation and support respiratory function. Early recognition and intervention are paramount in managing V/Q mismatches to avoid serious respiratory complications. Accurate interpretation of arterial blood gas analysis helps to identify the type and severity of any V/Q mismatch, guiding appropriate therapeutic decisions. This chapter thus underscores the vital importance of understanding ventilation-perfusion matching in the context of anesthetic practice, respiratory physiology and optimal patient care. The careful consideration of V/Q dynamics is essential for preventing and managing respiratory complications, ultimately contributing to improved patient outcomes. Effective management requires a comprehensive understanding of the underlying physiology, appropriate monitoring techniques, and the ability to tailor interventions to individual patient needs.

3.5 Diffusion Limitations

Efficient gas exchange hinges on the seamless transfer of oxygen and carbon dioxide across the alveolar-capillary membrane. This process, however, isn't always perfect. Several factors can impede this crucial exchange, resulting in a condition known as diffusion limitation. Understanding these limitations is vital for clinicians, particularly anesthesiologists, as they impact patient outcomes and guide treatment strategies.

The primary impediment to efficient diffusion is the thickness of the alveolar-capillary membrane itself. Increased thickness, often resulting from interstitial edema, fibrosis, or inflammation, increases the diffusion distance, thus slowing gas exchange. This is frequently observed in conditions like pulmonary edema, where fluid accumulation in the interstitial space creates a significant barrier. Imagine trying to push a ball through a thick layer of mud; the process is far slower and less efficient than pushing it through clear air. The same principle applies to gas exchange in the lungs.

Another major factor affecting diffusion is the surface area available for gas exchange. Emphysema, for instance, characterized by the destruction of alveolar walls, significantly reduces the total surface area available for gas exchange, leading to diffusion limitation. Think of it as reducing the number of windows in a house; less light (oxygen) can enter, hindering the overall process. Conversely, diseases such as pneumonia, characterized by alveolar inflammation and fluid filling, can also reduce the effective gas exchange surface area.

The partial pressure gradients of oxygen and carbon dioxide also play a critical role. A reduced alveolar partial pressure of oxygen (PaO2), as seen in high altitude or hypoventilation, directly impacts the driving force for oxygen diffusion. Similarly, an elevated alveolar partial pressure of carbon dioxide (PaCO2), often seen in hypercapnia, reduces the gradient for carbon dioxide elimination. The steeper the gradient, the faster the diffusion. A shallow gradient implies sluggish exchange, directly influencing arterial blood gas levels and ultimately, tissue oxygenation.

Diffusion capacity (DLCO), a measure of the lung's ability to transfer carbon dioxide across the alveolar-capillary membrane, provides a valuable clinical assessment tool. Reduced DLCO values indicate impaired diffusion capacity, suggesting underlying pathology such as interstitial lung disease or emphysema. Monitoring DLCO, alongside other respiratory parameters, enables clinicians to evaluate the severity of diffusion limitation and guide appropriate interventions.

The impact of anesthetic agents on diffusion is another important consideration. Some anesthetics can influence alveolar ventilation, leading to alterations in the partial pressure gradients and indirectly affecting diffusion. For instance, certain anesthetics can cause hypoventilation, leading to elevated PaCO2, thus reducing the driving force for carbon dioxide elimination. This is not a direct impact on the diffusion process itself but highlights the interconnectedness of respiratory mechanics and gas exchange.

Clinically, recognizing and managing diffusion limitation is crucial for optimizing patient outcomes. Early detection of underlying conditions, such as interstitial lung disease or emphysema, through thorough preoperative assessment and appropriate imaging techniques, allows for proactive management. In the perioperative setting, careful monitoring of arterial blood gases, including PaO2 and PaCO2, helps assess the adequacy of gas exchange. Supplemental oxygen therapy can help mitigate diffusion limitations by increasing the oxygen partial pressure gradient. In severe cases, mechanical ventilation might be necessary to maintain adequate oxygenation and carbon dioxide elimination. The goal is to ensure optimal gas exchange, prevent hypoxemia, and maintain adequate tissue oxygenation. Understanding the factors that contribute to diffusion limitations, and the strategies available to improve gas exchange, is pivotal for optimizing respiratory function. This knowledge is particularly relevant for anesthesiologists, who regularly manage patients with varying degrees of respiratory compromise. By recognizing and addressing these limitations, they can significantly improve patient outcomes and reduce the risk of postoperative complications. A thorough understanding of diffusion limitations is, therefore, not merely an academic pursuit; it's a cornerstone of safe and effective anesthetic practice and is crucial to promoting optimal pulmonary function in the perioperative period. Careful attention to detail and preemptive measures can significantly improve patient outcomes and reduce the risk of respiratory complications. The key lies in understanding the intricate interplay between various factors affecting gas exchange.

4 Control of Breathing

The rhythmic ebb and flow of respiration, seemingly effortless, is a complex interplay of neural commands and physiological responses. Understanding this intricate control system is crucial for any healthcare professional, particularly anesthesiologists, whose interventions can significantly impact this delicate balance. We'll delve into the central nervous system's role, focusing on the brainstem's respiratory centers and their intricate network of neuronal connections that generate the basic rhythm of breathing. These centers don't simply initiate breaths; they constantly adjust respiratory rate and depth to meet the body's ever-changing metabolic demands. Think of it as an orchestra conductor, meticulously coordinating the various instrumental sections. The dorsal respiratory group, for instance, plays a vital role in inspiration, driving the activity of the diaphragm and other inspiratory muscles. Meanwhile, the ventral respiratory group is more involved in expiration, particularly during periods of increased respiratory effort like exercise or respiratory distress. Their coordinated action ensures smooth transitions between inspiration and expiration, maintaining the rhythmic breathing pattern crucial for life. The pontine respiratory group, located in the pons, further refines this rhythm, modulating the output of the medullary centers, smoothing out the breathing pattern and preventing abrupt transitions. It's a dynamic, constantly adapting system, not a static, unchanging process.

Peripheral chemoreceptors, strategically positioned in the carotid and aortic bodies, act as the body's respiratory sensors. These specialized cells are exquisitely sensitive to changes in arterial blood gases—specifically, oxygen, carbon dioxide, and pH. A decrease in arterial oxygen levels, or an increase in carbon dioxide or hydrogen ions (leading to a drop in pH), triggers these chemoreceptors to send signals to the respiratory centers in the brainstem. This signal, relayed via the glossopharyngeal and vagus nerves, increases the activity of the respiratory centers, leading to an increase in respiratory rate and depth, effectively restoring arterial blood gas levels to their physiological set points. This intricate feedback loop is the body's way of ensuring adequate oxygenation and carbon dioxide removal, maintaining homeostasis.

However, the control of breathing isn't solely dependent on these chemical signals. Higher brain centers, such as the cerebral cortex and limbic system, also influence respiration. Voluntary control allows us to alter our breathing patterns consciously—holding our breath, for instance, or taking slow, deep breaths to calm ourselves. Emotional states can also significantly impact breathing. Stress and anxiety can lead to rapid, shallow breathing (hyperventilation), whereas relaxation and meditation often result in slower, deeper breaths. An understanding of these higher-level influences is essential when dealing with patients experiencing emotional distress or undergoing procedures that might trigger heightened anxiety. It impacts the patient's ability to cooperate during procedures.

The interaction between central and peripheral mechanisms is crucial. Imagine the situation: During strenuous exercise, your muscles demand more oxygen and produce more carbon dioxide. Peripheral chemoreceptors detect these changes, sending signals to the brainstem. Simultaneously, proprioceptors in the muscles and joints also send signals to the respiratory centers, signaling the increased metabolic demands. The brainstem integrates this information, adjusting respiratory rate and depth to meet the increased oxygen demand and eliminate the excess carbon dioxide. This coordinated response highlights the sophisticated interplay between various sensory inputs and the central respiratory control system. Understanding this integration is vital in predicting and managing respiratory responses to various stimuli and physiological states. The intricate feedback loops and complex interactions between different components, from the peripheral chemoreceptors to the higher brain centers, ensure the precision required to maintain optimal pulmonary function. The slightest disruption in this system can have profound consequences, highlighting the importance of a thorough understanding of respiratory control mechanisms in clinical practice.

4.1 Central Control Mechanisms

The rhythm of breathing, seemingly effortless, is orchestrated by a complex interplay of neural structures within the brainstem. This central control, residing primarily in the medulla oblongata and pons, isn't a simple on/off switch but a sophisticated system constantly adjusting ventilation to meet the body's metabolic demands. Respiratory centers, comprised of neuronal networks, generate the basic respiratory rhythm through intricate patterns of excitation and inhibition, a delicate dance of electrochemical signals. These rhythms are not static; they flexibly adapt to changing physiological circumstances.

Consider the intricate architecture of these respiratory centers. The dorsal respiratory group (DRG), located in the medulla, primarily controls inspiration. Its neurons activate the phrenic nerve, stimulating the diaphragm's contraction and initiating the inspiratory phase. Meanwhile, the ventral respiratory group (VRG), also medullary, plays a more complex role, influencing both inspiration and expiration, particularly during periods of increased respiratory demand, like exercise. Its neurons activate muscles involved in forceful breathing, such as the intercostal and abdominal muscles. This interplay ensures efficient gas exchange across a wide range of activities.

But the story extends beyond the medulla. The pontine respiratory group (PRG), residing in the pons, modulates the output from the medullary centers, refining the respiratory pattern. The PRG influences the transition between inspiration and expiration, smoothing out the breathing rhythm and preventing abrupt shifts in ventilation. This smoothing action is essential, ensuring a stable respiratory pattern even under dynamic conditions, preventing the jarring effects that would otherwise result from sudden changes in breathing rate and depth. Think of it as the fine-tuning system that prevents breathing from becoming erratic or excessively labored.

The system doesn't operate in isolation. Peripheral chemoreceptors, situated strategically in the carotid and aortic bodies, constantly monitor arterial blood gases, providing crucial feedback to the central controller. These sensory cells, highly sensitive to changes in oxygen partial pressure (PO2), carbon dioxide partial pressure (PCO2), and pH, send signals to the respiratory centers, adjusting ventilation to maintain homeostasis. A drop in PO2 or rise in PCO2, triggering a signal to increase respiratory rate and depth. This ensures sufficient oxygen uptake and carbon dioxide elimination. This feedback loop is vital in swiftly responding to environmental changes and maintaining consistent blood gas levels.

Integrating information from peripheral chemoreceptors is a significant aspect of the brain's regulatory role in breathing. The central chemoreceptors, located within the brainstem itself, are sensitive to changes in cerebrospinal fluid (CSF) PCO2 and pH. These chemoreceptors play a crucial role in maintaining acid-base balance and influencing ventilation based on CO2 levels in the CSF. A rise in PCO2 causes increased ventilation, compensating for increased acidity in the CSF. The brain's close proximity to these central chemoreceptors makes its response extremely rapid and crucial for homeostatic maintenance.

Furthermore, higher brain centers, such as the cerebral cortex and hypothalamus, can exert voluntary control over respiration. We can consciously alter our breathing rate and depth, exemplified by holding our breath or engaging in controlled breathing techniques. However, this conscious control is ultimately limited, as the medullary centers will override voluntary suppression of breathing when blood gas levels necessitate an immediate respiratory response. This protective mechanism prevents hypoxia or hypercapnia due to prolonged breath-holding.

Integrating this detailed understanding of central control mechanisms is paramount for clinicians and anesthesiologists. Conditions affecting the brainstem, such as stroke or trauma, can disrupt respiratory function, potentially leading to respiratory arrest. Similarly, anesthetic agents can depress central respiratory drive, necessitating careful monitoring and management of ventilation during anesthesia. This knowledge is therefore not just theoretical; it is directly applicable to patient safety and care. Understanding the fine interplay of signals, feedback loops, and integrating the conscious and unconscious control over breathing allows practitioners to predict, prevent, and effectively manage respiratory complications in the clinical setting. The complexity of these mechanisms underscores the importance of continuing education in this critical area of respiratory physiology. The delicate balance inherent in this system reveals the intricate mechanisms of the human body and the need for constant, precise regulation for optimal health. Therefore, a thorough comprehension of the central control mechanisms is pivotal for optimal patient management and avoiding serious complications.

4.2 Peripheral Chemoreceptors

Peripheral chemoreceptors, strategically located in the carotid bodies and aortic bodies, act as vital sentinels of the body's internal milieu. These small, highly vascularized structures continuously monitor the arterial blood, exquisitely sensitive to changes in oxygen partial pressure (PaO2), carbon dioxide partial pressure (PaCO2), and pH. Their primary function is to detect deviations from normal homeostasis and trigger compensatory adjustments in breathing, ensuring adequate oxygen delivery and carbon dioxide removal. This finely tuned system is crucial for survival, particularly in situations of hypoxia or hypercapnia.

The carotid bodies, nestled at the bifurcation of the common carotid arteries, receive a rich blood supply, ensuring continuous exposure to arterial blood. Their unique cellular architecture, featuring glomus cells that release neurotransmitters, allows for rapid signal transduction to the central nervous system. Afferent fibers from the carotid bodies travel through the glossopharyngeal nerve (IX), relaying information directly to the respiratory centers in the brainstem. Similarly, the aortic bodies, situated near the aortic arch, monitor arterial blood and transmit signals via the vagus nerve (X). Together, these chemoreceptors provide a redundant system, enhancing the body's capacity to respond to changes in blood gas composition.

Consider a scenario where PaO2 falls below its normal range. The glomus cells within the peripheral chemoreceptors detect this hypoxemia. This triggers a cascade of events: the glomus cells depolarize, releasing neurotransmitters, primarily dopamine, which activate afferent nerve fibers. The increased firing rate of these fibers transmits this crucial information to the respiratory centers in the medulla oblongata. The brainstem's respiratory control network, in response, initiates increased inspiratory drive, resulting in an elevation of respiratory rate and tidal volume – a rapid and effective compensatory mechanism to increase oxygen uptake. It's a testament to the body's remarkable ability to maintain homeostasis.

However, the chemoreceptors' response is not solely driven by oxygen levels. Elevated PaCO2 (hypercapnia) also significantly stimulates chemoreceptor activity. Hypercapnia leads to a decrease in blood pH (acidosis), which, along with elevated PaCO2, directly stimulates chemoreceptor discharge. This dual stimulation is particularly powerful, often resulting in a more pronounced ventilatory response than hypoxia alone. In fact, the ventilatory response to hypercapnia is often significantly more potent than that elicited by comparable degrees of hypoxia. This emphasizes the importance of carbon dioxide as a potent respiratory stimulant.

Understanding the interplay between oxygen and carbon dioxide sensing is critical in clinical practice. Patients with chronic obstructive pulmonary disease (COPD), for example, often exhibit chronically elevated PaCO2. In these individuals, the respiratory drive may become primarily dependent on hypoxic stimulation. Consequently, the administration of supplemental oxygen, while seemingly beneficial, can paradoxically suppress the already blunted hypoxic drive, potentially leading to respiratory depression. This highlights the complexities of managing respiratory failure in these patients and necessitates careful titration of oxygen therapy.

The sensitivity of peripheral chemoreceptors can be influenced by several factors, including age and underlying health conditions. For instance, with aging, the sensitivity to hypoxia may diminish. Similarly, certain medications, such as opioids and some anesthetic agents, can depress chemoreceptor activity, further compromising respiratory drive. Understanding these modifying factors is essential for providing safe and effective medical care. Such considerations are crucial during anesthesia, where respiratory depression is a common side effect of anesthetic agents. Careful monitoring of respiratory parameters is paramount in such settings.

Furthermore, the precise mechanisms involved in chemoreceptor function remain a subject of ongoing research. The interplay of various ion channels and signaling pathways within the glomus cells is complex and not fully elucidated. Ongoing studies continue to reveal new details about the intricate processes governing chemoreceptor sensitivity and function. For example, researchers are investigating the role of specific ion channels and receptors in regulating the release of neurotransmitters from glomus cells. This deeper understanding could potentially lead to new therapeutic targets for respiratory disorders.

In conclusion, peripheral chemoreceptors are essential components of the respiratory control system, acting as vital sensors of arterial blood gas composition and pH. Their precise and rapid responses to changes in oxygen, carbon dioxide, and pH ensure the maintenance of adequate gas exchange and are crucial for survival. A thorough understanding of their function is critical for clinicians in managing respiratory disorders, particularly in the context of anesthesia, where respiratory depression is a major concern. The complexities of chemoreceptor physiology provide ongoing opportunities for further research, potentially leading to advances in the treatment and management of respiratory diseases.

5 Anesthetic Effects on Respiration

Many anesthetic agents, regardless of their chemical structure, share a common effect: respiratory depression. This isn't simply a slowing of breathing; it's a complex interaction affecting various components of the respiratory system, from the central nervous system's control to the mechanics of gas exchange itself. Understanding these effects is crucial for safe anesthetic practice. The precise mechanism varies depending on the specific anesthetic used, however, the resulting impact frequently involves a decrease in respiratory drive, an increase in airway resistance, and a reduction in the responsiveness of the respiratory system to changes in arterial blood gases.

Opioids, for example, directly depress the respiratory center in the brainstem, resulting in slower and shallower breathing. Their influence extends beyond this central effect. Opioids can also affect the chemoreceptors, the body's sensors for blood oxygen and carbon dioxide levels, diminishing their sensitivity and reducing the body's natural response to hypoxia or hypercapnia. This blunting of the respiratory response necessitates careful monitoring and, if necessary, intervention to prevent hypoventilation and its associated complications. In contrast, inhaled anesthetics, while also causing respiratory depression, predominantly affect the respiratory muscles themselves, leading to decreased strength and efficiency of contraction. This can result in reduced tidal volume and minute ventilation.

The impact of anesthetic agents on respiratory mechanics is multifaceted. Airway resistance can increase due to bronchospasm or decreased muscle tone in the airway. Lung compliance, a measure of the lungs' ability to expand, may also be affected, making breathing more difficult. These changes can combine to significantly reduce the efficiency of gas exchange in the alveoli, leading to hypoxemia (low blood oxygen) and hypercapnia (high blood carbon dioxide). Careful attention must be paid to these factors during surgery and recovery, as even small changes can have significant consequences.

Effective management of respiratory depression during anesthesia is paramount. This involves a multifaceted approach that includes careful patient selection, titrating anesthetic doses meticulously, and employing sophisticated monitoring techniques. Preoperative assessment, including pulmonary function tests and a comprehensive medical history, is vital in identifying patients at increased risk of respiratory complications. During the procedure, continuous monitoring of respiratory rate, tidal volume, oxygen saturation, and end-tidal carbon dioxide levels (ETCO2) is essential.

Advanced monitoring techniques like capnography, which provides real-time measurement of ETCO2, are invaluable tools. Capnography not only allows for immediate detection of hypoventilation but also provides early warning signs of potential airway problems, such as disconnection or obstruction. These technologies enable prompt interventions, ranging from simple adjustments of anesthetic delivery to mechanical ventilation, ensuring the maintenance of adequate oxygenation and ventilation. Postoperative respiratory care is another critical aspect of managing respiratory complications.

The postoperative period often poses a significant risk of respiratory compromise, especially in patients with underlying lung disease or those who have undergone extensive surgical procedures. Aggressive respiratory support, including supplemental oxygen, incentive spirometry to encourage deep breathing, and early mobilization to promote lung expansion, are essential. Pain management is also crucial, as pain can inhibit deep breathing and coughing, increasing the risk of atelectasis (collapsed lung segments). A balanced approach integrating analgesic strategies and respiratory support maximizes patient recovery.

Understanding anesthetic effects on respiration isn't just about recognizing potential problems; it's about proactive risk mitigation. Thorough preoperative assessment, thoughtful anesthetic agent selection, meticulous titration of anesthetic doses, and vigilant monitoring are cornerstones of safe practice. The ultimate goal isn't merely to avoid respiratory depression, but to ensure that the patient's breathing is optimized throughout the perioperative period, minimizing the risk of complications and maximizing recovery.

The use of modern monitoring equipment, combined with an awareness of the subtle interactions between anesthetic agents and the respiratory system, allows anesthetists to provide the best possible respiratory care and promote safe and effective surgical outcomes. Furthermore, recognizing and addressing potential individual patient factors, such as age, obesity, and underlying pulmonary conditions, significantly improves the predictability and effectiveness of these interventions. Maintaining a comprehensive, personalized approach ensures the highest level of patient safety and minimizes the risk of respiratory complications. This involves not just monitoring vital signs, but also an understanding of the patient's respiratory response to the anesthetic and tailoring the management strategy accordingly.

5.1 Effects of Anesthetic Agents

The impact of anesthetic agents on respiration is multifaceted and clinically significant. Different agents exhibit varying degrees of respiratory depressant effects, primarily by affecting the central nervous system's respiratory control centers. This depression manifests as decreased respiratory rate, tidal volume, and ultimately, minute ventilation. Understanding these effects is paramount for safe anesthetic practice. Failure to properly manage these respiratory changes can lead to significant complications, including hypoxemia and hypercapnia.

Inhalational anesthetics, for instance, exert their effects by modulating neuronal excitability in the brainstem. Volatile agents like sevoflurane and desflurane, while effective, depress respiratory drive in a dose-dependent manner. This depression involves a reduction in both the sensitivity of chemoreceptors to changes in blood gas levels and the responsiveness of respiratory muscles to neural stimulation. This necessitates careful monitoring of respiratory parameters and proactive intervention when necessary. A patient's pre-existing respiratory condition will influence their susceptibility to these effects. For example, individuals with chronic obstructive pulmonary disease (COPD) may be more vulnerable to the respiratory depressant effects of even low doses of inhalational anesthetics.

Conversely, intravenous anesthetics, such as propofol and opioids, also significantly impact respiration, albeit through different mechanisms. Propofol, a commonly used sedative-hypnotic, depresses the respiratory centers directly, leading to a decrease in both respiratory rate and tidal volume. Opioids, potent analgesics frequently administered during anesthesia, induce respiratory depression by acting on opioid receptors in the brainstem, reducing the sensitivity to carbon dioxide and, consequently, the ventilatory response. Careful titration of these intravenous agents is crucial to minimize respiratory depression while maintaining adequate analgesia and sedation. This is achieved through vigilant monitoring of oxygen saturation, end-tidal carbon dioxide levels and arterial blood gas analysis as needed.

Furthermore, the interaction between anesthetic agents and other drugs, such as muscle relaxants and pre-operative medications, requires careful consideration. The combined effects of multiple respiratory depressants can be additive or synergistic, exacerbating respiratory depression. A clear understanding of the pharmacokinetic and pharmacodynamic properties of each agent is, therefore, essential for safe and effective anesthetic management. Close monitoring and judicious titration are critical to manage respiratory function and prevent adverse events.

The choice of anesthetic agent and technique should be tailored to the individual patient's characteristics and the nature of the surgical procedure. Patients with pre-existing respiratory disease or compromised pulmonary function require a particularly cautious approach, often involving a modified anesthetic technique to minimize respiratory depression and maintain optimal oxygenation. This might entail using lower doses of anesthetic agents or employing strategies such as positive pressure ventilation to support respiratory function. In such cases, individualized treatment plans are created to effectively address the unique challenges. The anesthetic plan must always consider the patient's overall health to assure a successful outcome.

Monitoring respiratory function during anesthesia is essential to detect and manage potential complications. Continuous monitoring of respiratory rate, tidal volume, oxygen saturation (SpO2), end-tidal carbon dioxide (EtCO2), and arterial blood gases (ABGs) provides valuable information about the patient's respiratory status. Capnography, which measures EtCO2, is a crucial tool for detecting hypoventilation and potential airway obstruction. Pulse oximetry, which measures SpO2, monitors oxygenation but does not directly assess ventilation, so it needs to be complemented by other monitoring techniques. Continuous monitoring helps detect early warning signs and facilitates prompt intervention. This vigilance is particularly important during and after the administration of anesthetic agents known for their respiratory depressant effects. Careful observation of the patient's clinical condition, in conjunction with these technological tools, assists in determining the patient's condition.

In summary, anesthetic agents significantly affect respiration, and understanding the specific mechanisms and clinical implications is vital for safe and effective anesthesia. Careful selection of agents, judicious titration, and meticulous monitoring are key elements in minimizing respiratory complications and maintaining optimal pulmonary function throughout the perioperative period. Continuous observation, attention to detail, and a thorough understanding of the patient's respiratory status are essential for ensuring patient safety. A multi-modal approach that incorporates various monitoring strategies, combined with the appropriate clinical judgment, is critical for the successful delivery of anesthesia and the management of potential respiratory complications.

5.2 Management of Respiratory Depression

Respiratory depression, a common complication of anesthesia, demands prompt and effective management. The underlying cause must be identified, which might involve a simple adjustment of anesthetic agent delivery or necessitate more intensive interventions. Failing to address it promptly can lead to hypoxia, hypercapnia, and potentially life-threatening consequences. Therefore, a structured approach is crucial.

Careful monitoring is paramount. Pulse oximetry, capnography, and arterial blood gas analysis provide essential data on oxygen saturation, carbon dioxide levels, and acid-base balance. These tools offer a real-time assessment of respiratory function, allowing for early detection of subtle changes indicative of worsening respiratory depression. Frequent observation of the patient's respiratory rate, rhythm, and effort provides additional valuable information. A thorough understanding of the baseline respiratory status is needed to identify deviations from the norm.

Initial management often involves reducing or discontinuing the causative anesthetic agent. This simple intervention can often reverse mild respiratory depression. Titrating volatile anesthetic agents downwards or switching to less respiratory-depressant agents may be effective. Opioids, frequently used in anesthesia, also contribute significantly to respiratory depression. Therefore, careful titration of opioid analgesics and the use of opioid antagonists, like naloxone, might be necessary. The decision to use these antagonists needs cautious consideration due to the potential for inducing opioid withdrawal symptoms.

Supporting ventilation becomes essential if respiratory depression is severe or unresponsive to initial measures. This may range from non-invasive techniques like continuous positive airway pressure (CPAP) or bilevel positive airway pressure (BiPAP) to intubation and mechanical ventilation. The choice of method depends on the severity of respiratory compromise and the patient's overall condition. CPAP offers support by maintaining positive airway pressure during both inspiration and expiration, preventing airway collapse. BiPAP adjusts the pressure delivered during inspiration and expiration separately, providing more precise control. Intubation secures the airway and allows for controlled ventilation, ensuring adequate oxygenation and carbon dioxide removal. Mechanical ventilation delivers precisely controlled breaths, adjusting volume, rate, and pressure based on individual needs.

Beyond the immediate management of respiratory depression, prophylactic measures play a critical role. A thorough preoperative assessment of the patient's respiratory health is essential. Identifying pre-existing conditions that might increase the risk of respiratory depression, such as COPD or sleep apnea, is vital. Such patients may require adjusted anesthetic techniques or closer monitoring. Moreover, optimizing the patient's preoperative respiratory status through measures such as smoking cessation and pulmonary physiotherapy enhances the resilience of their respiratory system and minimizes postoperative complications. Patients with a high risk should receive thorough preoperative pulmonary assessment and specific interventions to optimise their respiratory function before anaesthesia. The choice of anesthetic agents should also factor in their respiratory effects. Selecting agents with a lower propensity for respiratory depression should be preferred wherever possible. This careful selection helps minimize the risk of this complication. This careful approach helps to prevent respiratory depression, and lessens the burden on the patient. Careful planning and a thorough knowledge of various agents and their respective risks of causing respiratory depression can help prevent the complication. Postoperative respiratory care continues to play a crucial role in optimizing patient recovery. Early mobilization and deep breathing exercises are beneficial in restoring lung function and preventing atelectasis (collapse of lung tissue). This is particularly important for patients who have undergone major surgery or who are at a higher risk of postoperative respiratory complications. Physiotherapy is often used to help patients clear out the lungs and prevent the buildup of secretions that can further reduce their respiratory capacity. The use of incentive spirometry in the postoperative period plays an important role in helping patients improve their lung function. Pain management is another crucial component of postoperative respiratory care, as unrelieved pain can inhibit deep breathing and coughing, leading to complications. The team of healthcare professionals supporting the patient must be well versed in the use of various pharmacological and non-pharmacological interventions to optimally care for the patient. Regular monitoring of respiratory parameters and prompt intervention for any signs of deterioration are also key parts of successful postoperative care.

5.3 Monitoring Respiratory Function

Effective monitoring of respiratory function during anesthesia is paramount for patient safety and optimal outcomes. It's not just about reacting to problems; proactive monitoring allows for early detection of subtle changes, enabling timely intervention and preventing potentially catastrophic events. This involves a multi-faceted approach, integrating various tools and techniques to provide a comprehensive picture of the patient's respiratory status.

Accurate assessment begins with a thorough pre-operative evaluation. This includes a detailed history focusing on respiratory symptoms, known diseases, and smoking status. The physical examination assesses the patient's breathing pattern, looking for signs of distress, such as tachypnea or use of accessory muscles. Auscultation of the lungs provides critical information about breath sounds, identifying potential areas of consolidation or wheezing. Furthermore, basic pulmonary function testing, if feasible, can help predict potential risks and guide anesthetic management.

Continuous monitoring during the procedure is indispensable. Pulse oximetry provides a non-invasive, real-time assessment of oxygen saturation (SpO2), which although seemingly simple, is vital to detect hypoxemia. Capnography, measuring end-tidal carbon dioxide (EtCO2), offers a more direct measure of ventilation and the efficiency of CO2 elimination. Changes in EtCO2 can signal issues like hypoventilation, airway obstruction, or disconnections. Careful observation of the patient's chest movement, respiratory rate, and depth further supplements this data, allowing for early recognition of respiratory changes that might otherwise be missed.

Beyond these basic tools, more advanced modalities may be employed depending on the complexity of the case and the patient's condition. For instance, arterial blood gas analysis provides a comprehensive picture of oxygenation, ventilation, and acid-base balance. This invasive method, however, carries risks and is reserved for situations where less invasive monitoring proves insufficient. Similarly, esophageal pressure monitoring can aid in assessing respiratory mechanics, providing insights into the effectiveness of respiratory muscle function and potential complications. Transesophageal echocardiography may offer valuable information about cardiac function and its relationship to respiratory status, particularly in high-risk surgical procedures.

Interpreting the data obtained from these monitoring techniques requires a skilled approach. One should consider not only the absolute values, but also the trends and changes over time. A gradual decrease in SpO2, for instance, may indicate a developing hypoxemia, warranting timely intervention, even if the absolute value remains within the normal range. Similarly, a progressive increase in EtCO2 can point toward inadequate ventilation, while abrupt changes might suggest equipment malfunction or airway complications. The anesthesiologist's expertise is crucial in making informed clinical judgments, integrating data from multiple sources, and coordinating appropriate interventions.

Furthermore, remember that effective monitoring isn't just about technology; it also relies heavily on the anesthesiologist's clinical judgment and experience. Subtle cues, such as changes in patient behavior, heart rate, or skin color, may offer valuable clues regarding respiratory status. A comprehensive approach that combines technological monitoring with careful clinical observation yields the most reliable assessment. Ultimately, the goal is not just to detect respiratory problems but also to prevent them proactively through careful anesthetic management and close monitoring of physiological parameters. The seamless integration of technology and clinical judgment is essential for achieving optimal patient outcomes and preventing potentially life-threatening complications. Continuous education and a deep understanding of respiratory physiology are indispensable for anesthesiologists to fully appreciate the nuances of respiratory monitoring and effectively use this information to guide their clinical decisions. Therefore, maintaining a high degree of awareness and alertness is of utmost importance in ensuring patient safety throughout the procedure and recovery period. A successful outcome depends on an integrative, thoughtful approach to monitoring and managing respiratory function, incorporating both technological advancement and clinical intuition. The ultimate objective is to provide the safest and most effective anesthesia possible, considering every aspect of respiratory physiology and recognizing the subtle indicators that might signal developing problems. This approach, grounded in evidence-based practices and reinforced by continuous learning, is the hallmark of a skilled and responsible anesthesiologist. Effective monitoring is more than simply utilizing equipment; it's about understanding the physiology, integrating multiple data streams, and utilizing clinical acumen to provide the patient with the highest quality of care. The responsible practitioner recognizes the delicate balance between the various respiratory systems and ensures that every piece of data is assessed within the context of the individual patient's unique condition and response to the anesthetic. In conclusion, meticulous attention to respiratory monitoring and management is not merely a procedural necessity, but a critical aspect of ensuring patient safety and achieving optimal postoperative results.

6 Respiratory Disorders and Anesthesia

Managing anesthesia in patients with pre-existing respiratory conditions requires a nuanced understanding of both the disease process and the effects of anesthetic agents. Careful preoperative assessment is paramount, allowing for individualized anesthetic plans tailored to mitigate risks and optimize outcomes. Ignoring this crucial step can lead to potentially disastrous consequences.

For instance, patients with asthma present unique challenges. Bronchospasm, a life-threatening complication, can be triggered by various anesthetic agents, including volatile anesthetics and certain muscle relaxants. Therefore, meticulous selection of anesthetic medications is crucial, often favoring less bronchoconstricting agents. Preoperative optimization with inhaled bronchodilators and corticosteroids is also vital in preparing these patients for surgery. Intraoperative monitoring should focus on detecting early signs of bronchospasm, enabling prompt intervention with bronchodilators and potentially, mechanical ventilation.

Chronic obstructive pulmonary disease (COPD) presents a different, yet equally serious, set of concerns. These patients often exhibit decreased lung compliance and increased airway resistance, making adequate ventilation challenging during anesthesia. Careful attention should be paid to maintaining adequate oxygenation and avoiding excessive sedation that might compromise spontaneous breathing. Non-invasive ventilation strategies, such as CPAP or BiPAP, can be helpful both pre\item and postoperatively, aiding in maintaining oxygen saturation and reducing the work of breathing. The choice of anesthetic technique often leans towards regional anesthesia, whenever possible, to minimize the respiratory depression associated with general anesthesia.

Pneumonia adds another layer of complexity to anesthetic management. The inflammatory process within the lungs can significantly impair gas exchange, potentially leading to hypoxemia. Careful airway management and respiratory support are vital throughout the perioperative period. Preoperative chest physiotherapy can aid in mobilization of secretions, helping improve ventilation. Intraoperatively, close monitoring of oxygen saturation, arterial blood gases, and ventilator parameters are crucial. Postoperatively, aggressive respiratory support including airway clearance techniques, and early mobilization can minimize the risk of postoperative pulmonary complications.

Pulmonary embolism (PE) presents a life-threatening emergency, frequently encountered in the postoperative setting. Prompt diagnosis and treatment are critical. Prophylactic measures, such as early mobilization and the use of compression stockings, play a significant role in preventing

PE. Close monitoring for signs and symptoms of PE, such as shortness of breath, chest pain, and tachycardia is mandatory. If a PE is suspected, immediate imaging studies and treatment with anticoagulants are necessary. Anesthesiologists must be vigilant in detecting any indication of PE, as the consequences can be rapidly fatal.

Acute respiratory distress syndrome (ARDS) presents an extreme challenge. Characterized by severe hypoxemia, ARDS demands intensive respiratory support. Patients who develop ARDS post-surgery require meticulous management of fluid balance, ventilator settings, and meticulous monitoring. The ventilator strategy is often aimed at maximizing oxygen delivery while minimizing lung injury. Prone positioning can improve oxygenation, and other supportive measures might be necessary, depending on the severity of the condition. Mortality rates in patients with ARDS remain high, and careful planning and management are essential in minimizing risks. Successful anesthetic management in these diverse clinical scenarios requires a profound understanding of respiratory physiology, the pathophysiology of respiratory diseases, and the specific effects of anesthetic agents on pulmonary function. Close collaboration between anesthesiologists, pulmonologists, and other healthcare professionals is essential for optimal patient outcomes. By employing proactive strategies and individualized approaches, one can significantly improve patient safety and reduce the risk of perioperative respiratory complications. The key lies in careful assessment, meticulous planning, and vigilant monitoring throughout the perioperative period. This detailed and vigilant approach is not just a protocol; it is a commitment to patient safety and optimal outcomes. Every decision, from selecting an anesthetic agent to choosing ventilator settings, should be guided by a deep understanding of the patient's underlying respiratory condition and the potential interactions with anesthesia. This chapter has hopefully provided the tools to approach these critical situations effectively and safely. Remember, these guidelines aim to optimize patient care, and each case must be viewed and addressed according to its unique complexities and the physician's expertise.

6.1 Asthma and Anesthesia

Managing asthma in the perioperative setting presents unique challenges for anesthesiologists. The bronchospastic nature of asthma, triggered by various stimuli, requires careful consideration of anesthetic agents and techniques to minimize the risk of acute bronchospasm and perioperative complications. A thorough understanding of the patient's asthma history, including severity, frequency of exacerbations, and current medications, is paramount before proceeding with any anesthetic procedure. This preoperative assessment allows for the tailoring of anesthetic strategies to individual patient needs, optimizing the chances of a smooth and complication-free experience. Failure to do so could lead to severe adverse events.

Careful selection of anesthetic agents is vital. Potent inhalational agents like sevoflurane, while offering advantages in terms of speed of induction and emergence, can trigger bronchospasm in susceptible individuals. Therefore, the decision to use inhalational agents must be balanced against the potential risk of bronchospasm, and alternative options such as total intravenous anesthesia, using propofol and opioids, should be strongly considered for patients with a history of severe asthma or frequent exacerbations. This less invasive option can minimize the potential for triggering bronchospastic events during the procedure. This approach avoids many of the risks involved with inhalational anesthetics.

In addition to anesthetic agent selection, meticulous airway management is crucial. Pre-operative assessment should involve a thorough evaluation of the airway, taking into account any anatomical peculiarities or difficulties. Techniques like fiberoptic bronchoscopy can aid in difficult intubations, ensuring safe and effective airway control and preventing unexpected complications that could arise from difficult intubation attempts during the critical period. This is especially essential for patients with existing airway inflammation or hyper-reactivity. This ensures that there are minimal issues with the airways.

Maintaining adequate hydration is crucial throughout the perioperative period. Dehydration can worsen airway reactivity and increase the likelihood of bronchospasm. Intravenous fluids should be administered liberally, particularly in patients who are already dehydrated due to the effects of their asthma or who are receiving diuretics as part of their treatment regimen. Maintaining good hydration helps to ensure a consistent environment for the respiratory system, especially given that asthma is a highly reactive process that can be negatively impacted by dehydration. This simple measure plays a significant role in supporting the patient's overall respiratory function during the period of anesthesia and afterwards.

Bronchodilators play a vital role in managing asthma during anesthesia. Preoperative administration of short-acting beta-2 agonists, such as albuterol, can help to minimize airway reactivity and improve baseline pulmonary function. Maintaining this pretreatment and carefully monitoring for signs of bronchospasm helps minimize risks during the procedure. During surgery, inhaled bronchodilators can be readily administered if bronchospasm occurs, although their effectiveness can be sometimes blunted due to anesthetic induced changes in airway responsiveness. A multipronged approach using prophylactic measures and ready access to interventions is needed.

Postoperative respiratory care is just as important as perioperative management. Close monitoring of respiratory function, including respiratory rate, oxygen saturation, and the presence of any signs of wheezing or dyspnea, is necessary. Postoperative administration of bronchodilators and corticosteroids can help to prevent or treat any postoperative bronchospasm or inflammation. Early intervention can significantly reduce the length of hospitalization and improve patient outcomes, especially considering the risk of complications arising from post-operative respiratory issues in patients with asthma. Early recognition and immediate treatment are essential.

Finally, patient education plays a critical role in the successful management of asthma in the perioperative setting. Patients need to be informed about the risks associated with anesthesia and the measures that will be taken to minimize them. Clear communication can ease anxieties and increase the likelihood of compliance with pre-operative and post-operative instructions. This fosters a collaborative approach between the healthcare team and the patient, leading to better outcomes and reduces potential complications. This shared understanding creates a better environment for the patient.

6.2 COPD and Anesthesia

Chronic obstructive pulmonary disease (COPD) presents unique challenges during anesthesia, primarily due to its impact on lung mechanics and gas exchange. Patients with COPD often exhibit increased airway resistance, reduced lung compliance, and ventilation-perfusion mismatch, all factors significantly influencing their response to anesthetic agents. Therefore, a thorough preoperative assessment is crucial, including a detailed history focusing on symptom severity, exacerbations, and current treatments. This assessment should include pulmonary function testing (PFTs) to quantify the degree of airflow limitation and gas exchange impairment. A low FEV1/FVC ratio, indicative of obstructive disease, directly correlates with perioperative risk.

Careful attention must be paid to the patient's medication regimen. Bronchodilators, such as beta-agonists and anticholinergics, are typically continued perioperatively to optimize airway patency. Inhaled corticosteroids might be tapered, depending on the individual's condition and the surgical procedure's nature. The decision to continue or adjust these medications should be made on a case-by-case basis, considering the patient's clinical status and the potential interactions with anesthetic agents. This requires collaboration between the anesthesiologist, pulmonologist, and the patient's primary care physician. Close monitoring of the patient's response is mandatory.

The choice of anesthetic technique should prioritize minimizing respiratory depression. Regional anesthesia, when feasible, offers a valuable alternative to general anesthesia, particularly in patients with severe COPD. Regional techniques can lessen the need for high doses of sedatives and opioids and reduce the risk of post-operative respiratory complications. If general anesthesia is necessary, the selection of anesthetic agents should prioritize those with a relatively benign respiratory profile. Volatile agents like sevoflurane and desflurane, while potentially depressing respiration, offer better control over anesthetic depth and allow for quicker recovery.

Intraoperative management requires meticulous attention to respiratory parameters. Continuous monitoring of oxygen saturation, end-tidal carbon dioxide, and respiratory rate is essential. The use of capnography is particularly valuable in detecting hypoventilation or airway obstruction. Maintaining adequate oxygenation and avoiding hypoventilation are paramount. Positive end-expiratory pressure (PEEP) may be necessary to improve oxygenation and reduce atelectasis, but careful titration is crucial to avoid overdistension of already compromised alveoli.

Postoperative respiratory care is equally critical. Early mobilization, incentive spirometry, and the use of bronchodilators can significantly reduce the risk of postoperative pulmonary complications. Pain management should be tailored to minimize opioid-induced respiratory depression. Non-opioid analgesics, regional analgesia techniques, and multimodal analgesic strategies should be considered. Close monitoring of respiratory function, including frequent arterial blood gas analysis if necessary, continues until the patient's respiratory status has stabilized. Continuous positive airway pressure (CPAP) or non-invasive ventilation might be required for patients experiencing significant postoperative respiratory distress.

It is important to understand that managing anesthesia in COPD patients is a dynamic process demanding close observation and a flexible approach. The anesthesiologist's clinical judgment plays a crucial role in adapting the anesthetic plan to the patient's individual response. Careful attention to detail throughout the perioperative period—from preoperative assessment and medication optimization to meticulous intraoperative management and diligent postoperative care—is essential for ensuring optimal patient outcomes. A thorough understanding of the pathophysiology of COPD and its implications for respiratory function is paramount for achieving successful anesthetic management. The synergistic approach, including collaboration with other medical specialists such as pulmonologists and geriatricians, ensures the development of a well-defined and individualized anesthetic strategy.

The ultimate goal is to minimize the impact of anesthesia on the already compromised respiratory system, while providing adequate pain relief and surgical anesthesia. Regular reassessment and adjustments to the plan, based on the patient's ongoing clinical status, form an integral part of best practices. Remember that proactive measures, coupled with continuous monitoring and appropriate interventions, play a vital role in preventing complications and promoting a smooth postoperative recovery in COPD patients undergoing surgery. This patient population requires a multidisciplinary, nuanced approach that prioritizes both effective anesthesia and the preservation of respiratory function. Prognosis often hinges on careful pre-operative preparation and proactive post-operative care. Early identification of at-risk patients through thorough evaluation is paramount.

6.3 Pneumonia and Anesthesia

Pneumonia, a common lung infection, presents unique challenges during anesthesia. The inflammatory process itself, characterized by alveolar filling with exudate, significantly impairs gas exchange. This reduction in the functional alveolar surface area directly impacts oxygenation, potentially leading to hypoxemia, even under normal physiological conditions. The increased work of breathing, a consequence of the stiffening lung tissue and airway obstruction from secretions, further complicates the anesthetic process.

Careful preoperative assessment is paramount. A thorough history, including the severity and duration of the pneumonia, the presence of comorbidities like heart failure or COPD, and the patient's response to treatment, are all vital pieces of information. Chest radiography, pulse oximetry readings, and arterial blood gas analysis provide objective measurements of the extent of lung involvement and the patient's oxygenation status. This detailed assessment enables the anesthesiologist to tailor the anesthetic plan to the specific needs of the individual, minimizing risks and optimizing outcomes.

Positioning the patient appropriately is crucial for optimal ventilation. Consideration must be given to the patient's respiratory status to avoid any further impairment of their breathing mechanics. Proper positioning can help to maintain adequate lung expansion and improve gas exchange, especially important given the reduced lung compliance often associated with pneumonia. Strategies to prevent atelectasis, a condition that can severely compromise gas exchange, are particularly important during surgery. Careful monitoring and proactive measures to ensure adequate airway clearance are essential to minimize risks.

The choice of anesthetic agents requires careful consideration. Agents that cause minimal respiratory depression are preferred, while those that might further compromise respiratory function should be avoided or used with extreme caution, if necessary. A balanced approach, taking into account the patient's specific needs and the complexity of the surgical procedure is essential. In certain situations, regional anesthesia may offer advantages over general anesthesia, reducing the risks associated with general respiratory depression and related complications.

Intraoperative monitoring is critical during anesthesia for pneumonia patients. Continuous pulse oximetry and capnography provide real-time assessment of oxygenation and ventilation. Arterial blood gas analysis allows for more precise assessment of gas exchange and acid-base balance. These constant monitoring methods ensure that prompt intervention is possible should any deterioration in the patient's respiratory status occur.

Postoperative respiratory care is just as important as preoperative and intraoperative management. Early mobilization, incentive spirometry, and airway clearance techniques help to prevent atelectasis and pneumonia recurrence. Aggressive respiratory support, including mechanical ventilation if necessary, may be required in patients with severe respiratory compromise, allowing the body to recover without further complications. The close collaboration between anesthesiologists, surgeons, and respiratory therapists is imperative for successful management.

For patients with pneumonia undergoing surgery, a multifaceted approach is needed. A thorough evaluation of the patient's respiratory status before surgery is necessary for determining risk and planning a safe anesthetic approach, careful management during surgery, and meticulous postoperative respiratory care are all equally important in ensuring a successful outcome. The interplay between the inflammatory process, impaired gas exchange, and the effects of anesthesia necessitates a tailored approach to each individual patient's circumstances to minimize risks and enhance patient safety. Proactive measures can greatly reduce morbidity and mortality associated with pneumonia in surgical patients. The patient's overall health, the severity of the pneumonia, and the type of surgery must be considered in formulating an optimal anesthesia management plan. This individualized strategy minimizes potential complications and optimizes the patient's chance of recovery.

The use of bronchodilators and mucolytics may prove beneficial in improving airway patency. These medications can help to reduce airway resistance and facilitate the removal of secretions, thereby aiding in improving gas exchange. They can be administered prior to, during, or post-surgery, based on the patient's specific needs and the anesthesiologist's assessment. Careful consideration of potential drug interactions is vital, especially when multiple medications are used. Monitoring for any adverse effects is essential for ensuring patient safety.

Furthermore, attention to fluid balance is crucial in managing patients with pneumonia. The inflammatory response can lead to fluid shifts and pulmonary edema, potentially worsening respiratory function. Close monitoring of fluid intake and output is essential, ensuring that the patient's fluid status remains stable and that any fluid overload is avoided. Careful attention to intravenous fluid administration is vital in preventing or treating fluid imbalances, as it contributes towards respiratory stability.

In conclusion, the anesthetic management of patients with pneumonia requires a comprehensive and individualized approach. Preoperative assessment, careful selection of anesthetic agents, meticulous intraoperative monitoring, and proactive postoperative care are all critical elements that, when combined, can significantly reduce potential complications. This holistic approach, centered around preventing further respiratory compromise and optimizing pulmonary function, greatly improves the patient's chances for successful surgery and recovery.

6.4 Pulmonary Embolism and Anesthesia

Pulmonary embolism (PE), a life-threatening condition involving blockage of the pulmonary arteries by a thrombus, presents unique challenges during anesthesia. The presence of a PE significantly alters the patient's respiratory mechanics and hemodynamics, demanding careful consideration and proactive management. Failing to recognize and address these challenges can lead to catastrophic consequences, including cardiac arrest and death. Therefore, thorough preoperative assessment, meticulous intraoperative monitoring, and vigilant postoperative care are paramount.

Understanding the pathophysiology of PE is crucial. A thrombus, usually originating from deep vein thrombosis (DVT) in the lower extremities, travels through the venous system, eventually lodging in the pulmonary vasculature. This obstruction impedes blood flow to the lungs, causing ventilation-perfusion mismatch, hypoxia, and increased pulmonary vascular resistance. The severity of the impact depends on the size, number, and location of the emboli. Small, isolated emboli may be clinically silent, while massive PEs can lead to acute respiratory failure and circulatory collapse. The resultant increase in pulmonary vascular resistance increases the right ventricular afterload and can lead to right ventricular strain, failure, and even right ventricular rupture in extreme cases. This process acutely compromises oxygenation and can cascade into a myriad of other organ system failures.

Preoperative assessment for suspected or known PE is critical. A detailed history, including risk factors for DVT (e.g., recent surgery, prolonged immobility, malignancy, inherited thrombophilic conditions), is essential. Physical examination might reveal tachypnea, tachycardia, hypoxia, and potentially signs of right heart strain. Diagnostic imaging plays a pivotal role; a computed tomography pulmonary angiogram (CTPA) is the gold standard for diagnosing PE, providing detailed visualization of the pulmonary arteries. Other investigations, such as D-dimer tests and venous ultrasound scans, might be helpful in risk stratification.

Anesthetic management of patients with PE requires a multi-faceted approach. Maintaining adequate oxygenation is paramount, often necessitating supplemental oxygen and possibly mechanical ventilation. Careful hemodynamic monitoring is vital, utilizing invasive techniques (e.g., arterial line, central venous catheter) in most cases to continuously assess blood pressure, cardiac output, and central venous pressure. Fluid management is crucial; while volume resuscitation may be necessary in hypovolemic patients, excessive fluid administration can worsen right ventricular strain. Inotropic support may be required to maintain adequate cardiac output and blood pressure.

The choice of anesthetic agents needs careful consideration. Volatile anesthetics can depress myocardial contractility and potentially worsen right ventricular function, so agents with minimal cardiodepressant effects should be favored where possible. Regional anesthesia, if feasible, can reduce the need for general anesthesia and its associated respiratory and cardiovascular effects. Continuous monitoring of end-tidal carbon dioxide

(ETCO2) is crucial for detecting changes in ventilation and perfusion. Any unexpected increase in ETCO2 should alert the anesthesiologist to potential problems and necessitates prompt assessment.

Postoperative care must focus on preventing further thromboembolic events and optimizing respiratory function. Patients are typically maintained on anticoagulation therapy. Early mobilization and deep breathing exercises are encouraged to promote lung expansion and prevent atelectasis. Careful monitoring for signs and symptoms of recurrent PE is essential, and any clinical deterioration necessitates prompt investigation and management. The prevention of DVT is crucial; this involves strategies such as mechanical prophylaxis (e.g., graduated compression stockings, intermittent pneumatic compression devices) and pharmacologic prophylaxis (e.g., low-molecular-weight heparin).

In summary, the anesthetic management of patients with PE demands a high level of expertise and vigilance. Preoperative assessment and optimization, meticulous intraoperative monitoring, and proactive postoperative care are all crucial elements in minimizing risks and improving patient outcomes. A collaborative approach involving the anesthesiologist, surgeon, and intensivist is essential to ensure successful anesthetic management and prevent potentially life-threatening complications. The management of these patients can be challenging and always requires a thorough understanding of respiratory physiology, the hemodynamic effects of PE, and appropriate utilization of monitoring and supportive therapies. The use of evidence-based practices and a highly individualized approach, customized to each patient's clinical condition, remains the cornerstone of safe and effective anesthetic care in these complex scenarios.

6.5 ARDS and Anesthesia

Acute respiratory distress syndrome (ARDS) presents unique challenges during anesthesia. The hallmark of ARDS, diffuse alveolar damage leading to severe hypoxemia, necessitates a highly individualized anesthetic approach focused on minimizing further lung injury and optimizing oxygenation. Careful consideration of the patient's pre-existing comorbidities and the severity of their ARDS is paramount in developing a safe and effective anesthetic plan.

Preoperative assessment should be comprehensive, extending beyond the typical evaluation. A thorough review of the patient's medical history, including the specific cause and duration of their ARDS, is critical. Imaging studies, such as chest X-rays and computed tomography scans, provide valuable insights into the extent of lung injury and the presence of any complications like pneumothorax or pleural effusion. Pulmonary function tests, while challenging to interpret in ARDS, can offer some clues regarding lung mechanics and compliance. Understanding the patient's current respiratory support, including ventilator settings and oxygenation indices, is crucial for tailoring the anesthetic strategy. This meticulous approach allows for a more precise risk assessment and the selection of appropriate anesthetic techniques and medications.

The choice of anesthetic technique is heavily influenced by the patient's clinical status. Regional anesthesia, where feasible, offers the advantage of avoiding the respiratory depressant effects of general anesthesia. However, the severity of ARDS frequently necessitates general anesthesia for procedures requiring complete muscle relaxation or patient immobility. In such cases, meticulous attention must be paid to minimizing the duration of anesthesia and utilizing anesthetic agents known for their less pronounced respiratory depressant effects. Careful titration of volatile anesthetics, often combined with opioid analgesics, is essential to maintain adequate analgesia while avoiding excessive respiratory depression. Neuromuscular blockade, while sometimes necessary, should be employed judiciously, with close monitoring of neuromuscular function to prevent prolonged paralysis.

Maintaining optimal oxygenation during anesthesia is crucial in ARDS patients. This necessitates meticulous attention to ventilation strategies, including adjusting tidal volumes to minimize volutrauma and employing positive end-expiratory pressure (PEEP) to improve oxygenation. Careful monitoring of oxygen saturation, partial pressure of arterial oxygen (PaO2), and arterial carbon dioxide tension (PaCO2) is critical throughout the procedure. The use of advanced respiratory support techniques, such as high-frequency ventilation or extracorporeal membrane oxygenation (ECMO), may be considered for patients with severe hypoxemia despite optimal conventional ventilatory support. A proactive and vigilant approach to oxygen management is key to preventing further lung injury and improving patient outcomes.

Postoperative respiratory care is equally critical. Extubation should be carefully timed based on the patient's clinical condition and respiratory function, guided by careful monitoring and assessment. Continued respiratory support may be required postoperatively, with ongoing assessment and adjustments to ventilator settings as needed. Early mobilization, once clinically appropriate, can help prevent atelectasis and improve pulmonary function. Thorough physiotherapy and pulmonary rehabilitation play an important role in fostering optimal recovery, aiding in the restoration of respiratory function, and facilitating a return to baseline health. The overarching goal is to provide seamless care that seamlessly transitions the patient from the operating room into the critical care setting, maximizing their chances for a full recovery. This comprehensive and integrated approach is essential in managing the complex challenges presented by ARDS during the perioperative period. The key is constant vigilance, meticulous monitoring, and prompt action to improve outcomes for these critically ill patients. Success hinges on a collaborative effort across the surgical, anesthesia, and critical care teams.

7 Optimizing Pulmonary Function

Preoperative pulmonary assessment is crucial for identifying patients at high risk of postoperative pulmonary complications. Thorough history taking, focusing on smoking status, chronic respiratory illnesses like COPD or asthma, and any recent respiratory infections, provides a baseline understanding. A physical examination should include auscultation for abnormal breath sounds, noting any wheezes, crackles, or diminished breath sounds indicative of underlying pathology. Simple spirometry, measuring forced vital capacity (FVC) and forced expiratory volume in one second (FEV1), offers a quantifiable assessment of pulmonary function. A low FEV1/FVC ratio can signify obstructive lung disease, increasing the risk of postoperative respiratory distress. Patients with severely compromised pulmonary function might require further investigation, such as arterial blood gas analysis to determine oxygenation and ventilation status. Careful consideration of these factors allows for a tailored approach to anesthesia and perioperative management.

Postoperative respiratory care plays a vital role in preventing complications and ensuring a smooth recovery. Early mobilization and ambulation are essential to prevent atelectasis, a condition where the alveoli collapse. Deep breathing exercises and incentive spirometry encourage full lung expansion and prevent mucus accumulation. These simple, yet effective techniques help maintain adequate ventilation and oxygenation. Pain management is crucial; poorly managed postoperative pain can restrict chest wall movement, hindering effective breathing. Analgesics, including regional anesthesia techniques, should be implemented to optimize patient comfort and respiratory function. Continuous monitoring of respiratory parameters, including oxygen saturation, respiratory rate, and breath sounds, helps identify early warning signs of potential problems like hypoxemia or pneumonia. Prompt intervention based on these observations prevents the escalation of minor issues into serious complications. Continuous positive airway pressure (CPAP) or non-invasive ventilation may be employed to support ventilation in patients with compromised respiratory reserve.

The choice of anesthetic technique itself can influence postoperative respiratory function. Regional anesthesia, when feasible, often leads to improved postoperative respiratory outcomes compared to general anesthesia, minimizing respiratory depression and promoting faster recovery. The selection of anesthetic agents also merits careful consideration. Agents with known respiratory depressant effects should be used cautiously in patients with pre-existing respiratory disease. Careful titration of anesthetic agents and meticulous monitoring during the procedure are essential to avoid excessive respiratory depression. Postoperative analgesia plays a critical role;

appropriate pain control ensures adequate chest wall expansion and ventilation. The use of multimodal analgesia, combining various analgesic modalities, is increasingly favored to minimize opioid requirements and reduce the incidence of side effects such as respiratory depression.

Specific patient populations require a particularly vigilant approach to postoperative respiratory care. Patients undergoing major abdominal or thoracic surgery are at increased risk of atelectasis and pneumonia due to restricted chest wall movement and potential damage to lung tissue. Older patients are often more susceptible to respiratory complications due to age-related decline in pulmonary function and reduced reserve capacity. Patients with pre-existing respiratory conditions such as COPD, asthma, or cystic fibrosis require close monitoring and tailored strategies to prevent exacerbations. For instance, patients with asthma might benefit from prophylactic bronchodilator therapy in the postoperative period. For patients with COPD, careful attention should be paid to maintaining adequate oxygenation and minimizing respiratory drive depression from medications.

Optimizing pulmonary function demands a multifaceted approach encompassing preoperative assessment, judicious anesthetic management, and meticulous postoperative care. This involves a holistic understanding of respiratory mechanics, gas exchange, and the patient's specific risk factors. Careful consideration of these factors, coupled with the implementation of evidence-based strategies, significantly enhances the patient's chances of a safe and efficient recovery. The ultimate goal is to minimize the risk of postoperative pulmonary complications, ensuring optimal respiratory function and a swift return to normal activity. This proactive approach underscores the significance of integrating comprehensive respiratory management into the overall surgical care plan. Through careful assessment, tailored anesthetic techniques, and diligent postoperative monitoring, we can optimize patient outcomes and improve their quality of life. Effective communication amongst the surgical team, including anesthesiologists, nurses, and respiratory therapists, is essential for coordinated care and successful pulmonary function optimization.

7.1 Preoperative Pulmonary Assessment

A thorough preoperative pulmonary assessment is crucial for minimizing postoperative respiratory complications. It involves a detailed history focusing on current and past respiratory illnesses, including frequency and severity of symptoms like cough, sputum production, dyspnea, and wheezing. The patient's smoking history, including pack-years and cessation status, is paramount, as smoking significantly increases the risk of postoperative pulmonary complications. This information paints a picture of the patient's baseline respiratory health and informs the subsequent parts of the evaluation.

Next, a physical examination is vital. This involves auscultation of the lungs to identify abnormal breath sounds such as wheezes, crackles, or diminished breath sounds, indicators of underlying respiratory disease. We must pay close attention to the patient's respiratory rate, rhythm, and effort. Cyanosis, clubbing of the fingers, or use of accessory muscles for breathing should trigger further investigation, potentially highlighting compromised respiratory function. Careful observation and detailed notation are key.

Pulmonary function testing (PFTs) provides objective measurements of respiratory function. Spirometry, measuring forced expiratory volume in one second (FEV1) and forced vital capacity (FVC), assesses the degree of airway obstruction. Other tests, such as diffusing capacity of the lung for carbon monoxide (DLCO), may be indicated to assess gas exchange efficiency. The results of these tests, along with the patient's history and physical examination, allow us to quantitatively assess their respiratory status and accurately stratify their risk of postoperative pulmonary complications. Interpreting these results requires a nuanced understanding of normal values and age-related variations.

Chest radiography is a commonly used imaging modality to visualize the lungs and identify any abnormalities such as infiltrates, effusions, or masses. While not always necessary in low-risk patients, it is valuable for those with a concerning history or physical examination findings, adding another layer to our assessment. A chest x-ray can help us visualize the extent of any underlying disease and further clarify the patient's suitability for surgery.

Beyond the standard tests, we must consider factors specific to the patient and the planned procedure. The type of surgery, its anticipated duration, and the patient's overall health, including the presence of comorbidities such as cardiac or neurological disease, influence the risk profile. A patient undergoing a major abdominal surgery will face different respiratory challenges than one having minor outpatient procedure. A comprehensive preoperative evaluation, therefore, should consider this context.

Finally, the results of the assessment should inform the development of a perioperative management plan to mitigate potential respiratory risks. This may include pre-operative physiotherapy to improve respiratory muscle strength, cessation of smoking, treatment of any identified infections, or the optimization of the patient's medical condition. Moreover, the anesthesiologist should be thoroughly informed of all findings to enable appropriate anesthetic management choices. Collaborating with the surgical team and other healthcare providers to tailor treatment strategies guarantees holistic care and improved patient outcomes. Remember, thorough preoperative assessment is not just a protocol; it's a crucial step in safeguarding patient safety and promoting successful surgical outcomes. It requires careful consideration, meticulous attention to detail, and a collaborative approach to create a personalized care plan which ultimately reduces the potential of respiratory complications post-surgery. The ultimate goal is to ensure safe and effective anesthetic management tailored to each individual's unique respiratory profile. This proactive approach helps minimize risks and enables the patient to recover smoothly, prioritizing their overall well-being.

7.2 Postoperative Respiratory Care

Early mobilization is key. Getting patients out of bed and moving around, even short distances, soon after surgery significantly reduces the risk of atelectasis and pneumonia. Encourage deep breathing exercises and coughing to help clear secretions. Pain management is crucial here; uncontrolled pain can inhibit deep breathing and coughing, hindering recovery. Physiotherapy input is invaluable; a respiratory physiotherapist can tailor exercises to the individual patient, ensuring comfort and effectiveness. They'll also teach techniques for effective airway clearance.

Monitoring vital signs, including oxygen saturation, respiratory rate, and heart rate, is paramount. Close observation allows for early detection of any respiratory distress, enabling timely intervention. Pulse oximetry provides a continuous assessment of oxygen levels, alerting clinicians to any desaturation. Regular chest auscultation helps identify the presence of crackles or wheezes, indicating possible pneumonia or fluid accumulation. Arterial blood gas analysis may be necessary to provide a comprehensive assessment of oxygenation and ventilation.

Incentive spirometry is a simple yet effective technique to encourage deep breathing. It helps expand the lungs, improving gas exchange and preventing atelectasis. Patients should be instructed on proper use, ensuring correct inhalation technique and holding their breath for the recommended duration. Regular use, ideally every hour while awake, maximizes its benefit. Visual aids and patient education materials can improve adherence and understanding.

Secretion management is vital for preventing airway obstruction and infection. Techniques such as postural drainage and chest physiotherapy help mobilize secretions. Suctioning may be required if secretions are thick or excessive. Humidification of inspired air thins secretions, facilitating their removal. Remember, diligent attention to hydration is essential for keeping secretions fluid and easily expectorated. The patient's hydration status must be monitored closely.

Maintaining adequate hydration is crucial for optimal respiratory function. Dehydration thickens secretions, making them harder to clear, increasing the risk of infection. Monitoring fluid intake and output helps assess the patient's hydration status. Intravenous fluids may be necessary if oral intake is insufficient. Careful attention to electrolyte balance is also important, as imbalances can affect respiratory muscle function. Regular monitoring of electrolyte levels is important, with adjustments made as needed.

Pain management plays a crucial role in postoperative respiratory care. Uncontrolled pain can hinder deep breathing, coughing, and mobilization. Adequate analgesia is essential to allow the patient to participate fully in respiratory exercises and mobilization. A multimodal approach, combining different analgesic modalities, may be the most effective. Regular pain assessments and adjustments to the pain management plan are needed to maintain patient comfort and facilitate optimal respiratory function. Effective communication between the patient and the healthcare team is central to this process.

Close monitoring for signs of respiratory complications, such as increased respiratory rate, shortness of breath, decreased oxygen saturation, or the appearance of new crackles or wheezes, is essential. Prompt detection and management of these complications can prevent serious deterioration. Early intervention with supplemental oxygen, bronchodilators, or antibiotics, if needed, improves outcomes. Regular communication between the nursing staff, respiratory therapists, and physicians ensures a coordinated approach to managing potential respiratory problems. The patient's response to interventions needs continuous review.

Postoperative respiratory care is not a static process, but rather a dynamic interaction between the patient, their physiology, and the healthcare team. It requires ongoing assessment, adjustment of treatment plans, and a commitment to patient education and empowerment. Collaboration between different healthcare professionals is fundamental, ensuring that all aspects of respiratory care are addressed holistically. This patient-centered approach is vital for optimizing respiratory function and promoting a safe and efficient recovery. The goal is always to achieve optimal pulmonary function and minimize the risk of postoperative respiratory complications. Open communication with the patient and family helps ensure compliance with the treatment plan, fostering a more effective and less stressful postoperative recovery.

www.ingramcontent.com/pod-product-compliance
Lightning Source LLC
LaVergne TN
LVHW020237210926
848481LV00016B/2349
9798349296086